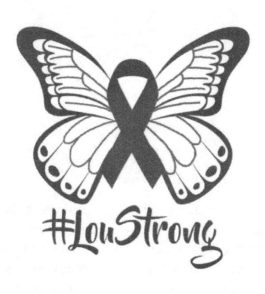

ISBN: 978-1-312-65631-4

First published in the United States in 2023.
Mahi Bay, LLC
Marietta, Ohio

Cover Design by Chad Wittekind
Printed in the United States of America
Distributed in the United States by Mahi Bay, LLC

I'M not FINE

But I'm Surviving Cancer

I will be forever humbled and grateful to all of my family and friends who have supported and encouraged me during my journey and continue to do so. Thank you for always being there for me without question. You truly brighten my spirits. I love you all so very much.

I would not be where I am today without my incredible medical team. Thank you for the compassion, patience and expertise you give to, not just me, but all of your patients, each and every day. I hold so much respect and admiration for you.

I am fully aware of just how lucky I am to have all of you in my life and thank God for you every single night. As my mother would say: "my cup runneth over".

For my husband, who I undoubtedly would not have made it through this journey without. My strength, my rock, my person. Thank you for being the amazing man you are, for loving me unconditionally and for taking care of me with patience and grace. I love you three thousand, forever and always.

Foreward

by Shawn Modesitt

I first met my wife 19 years ago and immediately had an overwhelming connection to her, so much so, that we fell in love and got married. Leigh Ann is a strong gentle soul that is rooted in family. Her enjoyment comes from others enjoyment. I immediately noticed her carefree aura and fun-loving nature. The things that are important to my wife are family, experiences, friendship, and giving to others. She frequently puts the needs of others ahead of her own and gets fulfillment from these acts. My wife is very artistic and finds great pleasure in drawings, crafting and photography. Pictures have always been extremely important; they are a reminder and a glimpse into special times with special people. Her role models have always been her Grandparents and Mother, very strong, loving, committed, and self-reliant individuals. It is evident she gets her determination from them. I always say she is the strongest person I know.

My wife and I have been through everything together. I have never left her side no matter how difficult the situation. We have spent numerous nights in the hospital together sharing meals, watching movies, holding hands during treatments, and making sure that we supported each other. Our marriage is a partnership, what one goes through the other also goes through. It's important that I never l left her side, and in that, she has never left mine either. We always find strength in each other: when one can't anymore, the other makes sure they can. My wife often refers to me as her "rock", I think she is the unbreakable force in our marriage that inspires me continually.

My wife has been through many journeys in her diagnosis and treatments. Her inquisitive nature lends itself to many hours of research on her cancer, treatments, and cutting-edge advancements. She frequently attends seminars, events, and virtual treatment advancement webinars. Knowing what to expect eases the stress of doubt and fear. She has immersed herself in her cancer community creating professional and personal relationships. She often gives counsel to others on their own journey providing that emotional relatability that is so desperately needed. These relationships have created a tribe that fills a void that only people that have heard the phrase "you have cancer" can understand. The support these friends provide is very personal, and one I think they only really understand. Even more importantly, the tribe and close friends provide an outlet of fun and normalcy in a not normal situation.

I found an array of emotions and reflections reading about my wife's journey. Her book does an outstanding job conveying what it means to navigate the cancer rollercoaster. The book takes you on the whirlwind of emotions and questions that all cancer patients go through. Through milestones and setbacks, she gives an accurate and emotional reflection of every part of her journey over the last four years. I was amazed how the book touched me. After all, I have been here since the beginning, how could I not understand everything she is feeling? I couldn't put it down. I think anyone who has been touched by cancer will relate to my wife's continuing journey. I am amazed everyday by her strength to overcome and her ambition to help others.

Prologue

2018 - The Year Before it All Changed

You should be here. This song was released the day my Bubba passed away. One of my biggest supporters in this world and she was gone too soon. It is March 23, 2018, and as an early birthday present, I have just met Cole Swindell. As he sings this song in a small VIP area to a select few, I am bawling like a baby. I can't help myself. If people are looking at me, I don't notice because all I can think of is how desperately I miss my grandma. My husband, Shawn, holds me tight, allowing me to get it all out, although I am positive that I am embarrassing him. He stands five feet ten inches with baby blue eyes and a thick head of sandy brown hair, though his trimmed facial hair was slowly becoming grey. Although I had a brief moment of sadness over the aforementioned song, I am still giddy with excitement this evening. We are able to gather autographs as well as amazing photographs to commemorate this event. Tonight, we are in the pit by the stage, singing along to every word. My husband has his arm around my waist as we sway along to the music. It is so loud we can't hear each other talk but every so often he will lean over to kiss my forehead and I will give him a sheepish smile. I can feel the boom of the speakers echoing inside my chest. It's exhilarating. The crowd is singing and cheering along, only becoming louder as the momentum increases with each new artist arriving on the stage. How lucky are we to have this experience?

Shawn and I have been going to concerts since we first began dating. So far, in the last month, we have attended two musical performances. We were able to meet three of our favorite artists this year. I have always enjoyed music of all genres. It has been my escape. Often an emotional release. A reason to laugh when I attempt a dance move that, most likely, I just created. A tender moment with my husband dancing in the kitchen as he serenades the words to me.

A couple months later, in May, as I sit in an auditorium packed with a multitude of other parents, I am filled with so many emotions. My son is graduating high school at the top of his class. The day he was born, he instantly became my everything – my whole world. The last two years of high school he also has been attending a local community college. Due to this opportunity, he was able to graduate with his Associates Degree a couple weeks ago, prior to finishing high school. As I sit here waiting for his name to be called, camera ready to capture this special moment, I try to make sense of how the last eighteen years have flown by so quickly. I remember holding him on my chest, taking in his baby scent, the day he took his first steps and the first time he looked at me with those big brown eyes with the most precious smile and called me Mommy. His bright blonde hair had grown darker over the years and he now wore navy blue plastic rectangular glasses, but his infectious smile and those amazing dimples haven't changed a bit. As I watch him walk down the aisle past me, tears start to trickle down my cheek. My heart is beaming with pride for the young man he has become. I can't wait to discover all the wonderful things I know he will do in the future.

The summer seemed to disappear in a blink of an eye. Caleb had been accepted to several colleges but eventually decided on the University of Akron. The school was only a couple hours away from our hometown of Marietta, Ohio. Given one of his prospective schools was in Nova Scotia, Canada, I was happy to have him closer to home. My mother and I spent days purchasing all of the items he may need at school (and then some). We canned soups, salsa and vegetables for him to be able to warm up in his dorm room. We live on a small farm with a large garden where fresh produce is abundant. I have always been that mom who worries about everything. People often warned me that I would never understand the unconditional love and constant worry that comes with being a parent until I had a child of my own. I grasped that concept the first time I looked at my baby boy. That concern only grew stronger the older he got as he started driving, going out and coming home later. Caleb started a vegan diet in high school and at that time there were few viable options at the college. I wanted to ensure that he had plenty of food in his dorm from home that he could eat, if needed. This, of course, would also result in me making sure he went back to school with an overload of dinners I prepared for him every time he came home to visit. I love to cook and bake. It has always been one of my greatest passions in life. My son took an interest in cooking early on in his childhood and we spent an extensive amount of time together in the kitchen. Some of my fondest memories are of him creating his own recipes as a little boy and surprising us with dinner. As he got older, he would look up fancy recipes online and prepare them for us for supper. I knew in my head that he was an amazing, smart, talented young man who was going to thrive in college, but my heart wanted him to stay home forever. When August was coming to an end, an entourage of his family drove the two hours to Akron in a convoy of cars to move him in to his new dorm room. We spent the day hanging photos of his family and friends on the wall and making sure his cabinets and fridge were full of food. After everyone departed, I was clinging on to one last night with just the two of us. We went out to dinner, discovered new stores around town and stayed up talking under the dim lights of a hotel room. I was so excited for all of his new adventures but the mom in me was still holding on to my little boy. As we parted ways the following day, I spent the next two hours driving home alone, listening to the playlist of songs on a CD that he had created a few years ago for my birthday. Some of them would make me smile, conjuring up a memory, others would make the tears overflow. My whole life up to this point was taking care of him and I had to learn how to let go because I knew he was going to go out there and try to change the world. He was majoring in social work and had made it his mission to help those who were neglected the most in life. In order to reduce my worry, he was diligent in checking in with me via text or a call daily....for the most part.

Shawn and I were now officially empty nesters. At the age of thirty-seven, I found myself trying to adapt to this life-changing moment. The last eighteen years have revolved around my child. School events, sports games, birthday parties, music concerts and all the other wonderful things that come with raising a child. I missed lying in bed at night listening to him softly strum his guitar or practice the violin. He was a talented musician who taught himself how to play a plethora of instruments. For years, I had drifted off to sleep to the sound of his guitar. Nighttime was now silent.

I am one of those people who do better in life when I stay busy. Less time for my head to wander and worry about things I am unable to control. Easier said than done. Even learning to cook for only two people was challenging. I threw myself into my work. I had been employed for a local attorney for over a decade. My main responsibility was filing estates with the Court and guiding the beneficiaries through the process which could take up to a year to finalize. I loved my job. I was able to form relationships with my clients and help them in their time of grieving. I have known my boss since I was a little girl. He is small in stature with snow white hair on his face and what little he had left on his head. He was generous and kind, the type of person everyone appreciated. Over the years, he had become another fatherly figure in my life with whom I had the utmost respect for and cherished dearly.

Shawn and I stayed busy taking trips, enjoying fall events, attending a few more concerts and learning to slow down. He also took me to my first golf tournament where I was lucky enough to obtain a photo with one of my favorite golfers. We were just beginning to chart out future plans to travel, excited to cross off destinations on our bucket list.

We were unaware of how much our lives were about to change...

1

Sept. 2018 - Something's Wrong

Three years ago, I was still having a hard time adjusting to daily life after losing two of my grandparents the previous year, both of whom I had been extremely close to. My husband decided to take me away on a trip to get me out of town for a few days. I am normally a spreadsheet loving, obsessive compulsive, researching planner and this trip was a spur of the moment getaway to a place we had never visited, randomly chosen from a Google search. We settled on Destin, Florida, known as the "World's Luckiest Fishing Village" located on the panhandle. Normally, all of the uncertainty would have overwhelmed me, but my soul was still wounded and I didn't have the energy to stress about it. From the first moment we got there, we fell in love with everything about the area. The beaches were covered in soft white sand that felt like powder in between my toes. That part of the gulf is known as the Emerald Coast due to the indescribable waters that vary in color from mint green to teal blue to the most amazing shade of emerald. The water is as clear as glass inviting you to get lost gazing out in to it for hours. I would much rather be on the water than sitting on a beach. Destin allows me to do both. My favorite part is relaxing on a pontoon at Crab Island where I get overly giddy when I see a dolphin. I love the feel of the breeze blowing against my face when we go full speed on a jet ski. That trip was everything that I needed to recharge and from then on, we tried to visit the area as often as possible.

So far this year, we had been lucky enough to visit Destin in April and we took Caleb and one of his friends with us in May after his graduation. It is now September and my mom, Jean, and her husband, Al, have joined us for part of our vacation. My mother is beautiful. She has thick dark blonde hair moving on to grey, hazel green eyes that match mine, glasses with just a hint of purple and a metabolism that would make anyone envy her thin figure. She is caring, gentle, a stubborn hard worker and is always there for me without question. Al started dating my mom when I started high school which eventually led to marriage and our family moving from town out to the farm. I grew to love this luxury of being able to walk out on my deck to be surrounded by natures beauty. Eventually, I would purchase Al's father's house on the farm and still reside there to this day. Al accepted me as his daughter from day one and has shown me nothing but unconditional love since we first met. He is a quiet, hardworking man with short brown hair and thin wired glasses, who always sees the best in someone and the beauty in life. My mother holds a special place in her heart for the beach, as it is something that still keeps my grandmother alive in her heart. Although she will always prefer the shores of Ocean City, New Jersey, they quickly fell in love with Destin and vowed to come back every fall with us. We had scheduled a fishing trip with a captain we had come to know well and considered a friend. Shawn has always been an avid fly fisherman and was initially unsure of how he may feel about not using a fly rod offshore. He quickly realized he enjoyed the thrill of reeling in the saltwater gulf fish. Each trip down we did an offshore fishing trip together, then he often went out on a fly-fishing trip on his own. It takes a while to arrive at a good fishing spot but the ride there is exhilarating. I am surrounded by nothing but breathtaking emerald waters, wind blowing my hair and the up and down bounce of the boat catching each wave. On occasion, an enormous leatherneck sea turtle will come by or an awe-inspiring pod of dolphins would swim up to the boat. Although the fisherman aren't fans of them, due to the fact they scare away the fish, I would always insist the guys stop anyway so I could gaze at them. They would indulge me every time, floating around for a short while, allowing me to get lost in the magic of my surroundings. The gulf is plentiful of fish, including red and mingo snapper, grouper, amberjack, mahi mahi and redfish, as well as many other species. When we first began fishing, the guys would help me reel in my catch, but they quickly stopped assisting me as I became really good at doing it on my own. Sometimes I would reel in larger fish – and more fish – than Shawn which was always fun to brag about later that evening. We would keep what was in season, just enough to eat for the week, as we wouldn't be able to transport any excess fish back to Ohio easily. There are many restaurants that do what they call 'hook and cooks' where you take your daily catch in for them to prepare it. Our meal would come out on giant wood cutting boards, towering with different preparations of our fish, typically fried, blackened and grilled. Surrounding the fish was always potatoes or grits, green beans or asparagus, corn on the cob with warm butter melted over it, and hushpuppies. Fellow diners would stop eating to gawk at our masterpiece as it was brought to our table. As we had started taking family and friends down there with us by this point, the dinner would be enough for all of us, plus plenty of food to take back to the condo to warm up for dinner over the next couple of nights.

On this fishing trip, however, I didn't feel quite right. I have never had an issue getting sea sick so it wasn't anything like that. I was lightheaded and weak. I spent a lot of time resting in the marine bean bag at the back of the boat that I had determined was the most comfortable, relaxing chair ever invented. Unfortunately, we did not catch a lot of fish that day, but we did get some mingo snappers to keep, which was our favorite fried fish anyway. My parents weren't sure about going on a boat off shore so they met us at the marina dock at the end of the excursion. When we arrived, my mom immediately asked if I was okay, concerned that I didn't look well. I assured her I was fine and we went back to the condo to freshen up for dinner. Within minutes, I became extremely cold and started shaking uncontrollably. I crawled into bed and threw every blanket we had over top me. At some point, someone suggested I take a hot shower. The steaming water poured over me and, as wonderful as it felt, I still could not stop shivering. My mom called my brother, who is a nurse practitioner, and he advised her to get some Pedialyte in me as I may be dehydrated. It was a long, miserable evening. Shawn held me all night to try to warm my body and calm my quivers. My mom was distraught with worry and they were due to fly back to Ohio the next morning. I was on the water often and had never had anything like this happen to me before so I was growing slightly concerned. I stayed in bed the next day to rest and felt better the following one. We enjoyed our last day in Destin and then we, too, flew back home and didn't give my night of freezing another thought.

Fast forward a couple of months to December. A purple rash began taking over my toes. It started off small then quickly spread to all of my toes and started moving to the tops of my feet. Eventually, I gave in and went to see my Dermatologist. I work in an older building that doesn't heat well so we were always chilly in the winter. My doctor diagnosed me with Chillblains, which is a painful inflammation in blood vessels due to exposure to cold. She said it could be an autoimmune disease such as lupus and, if I wanted to, I could get some blood work done to rule that out. Not wanting to deal with all of that, we settled on wearing thicker socks at work and obtaining a small heater to put under my desk. If they didn't clear up in a couple weeks, I would come back for labs. I would go on to think back on this appointment often down the road and how things could have turned out differently if I would have given in to the bloodwork that day.

A few days later, Shawn had a Christmas party for work in Columbus, Ohio, which is about two hours away, so we decided to make the most of it and stay for the weekend. After the party, we went with some friends to Top Golf, where we all had a great time hitting golf balls. I scored a second-place finish, outscored only by my husband. We finished the evening by going to see the Chinese Dragon Lights. I love everything about this experience. I have always been creatively artistic and there is just something about the beauty in all of the colors and the art of the lights that gets me excited. And of course, the photos. Shawn indulges me by taking selfies in front of all the fascinating works of art beaming with light. I then rush straight to the noodle bowl booth. It is cold outside and the warm broth rushes through my body as I savor every spoonful of the long, curly pasta. Ramen and pho are at the top of my favorite foods list so I look forward to this feast every year. The next day we head over to an outdoor mall area to do some shopping before we drive back home. We were going to miss the turn in, so Shawn slammed on the breaks and did a sharp right turn into the parking lot. I screamed in agony. In an instant, I felt a pain unlike I had ever experienced in my back. Shawn was in a panic. I felt like I couldn't catch my breath. We were both trying to make sense of what happened in that moment. The week before, I was carrying groceries into the house, being far too stubborn to make more than one trip, and the handle of the screen door closed on me, hitting me right on my spine. My back had been a little sore since then but I hadn't really thought too much about it as I assumed it was simply a bruise that would slowly go away. Shawn suggested we head home immediately but I insisted I was fine and needed to get some Christmas shopping done. Inevitably, after only one store, we headed back to Marietta.

I had no idea just how drastically my life was about to change.

2

Powering through

The next couple of days I continued to go to work during the day and tried to recover in bed in the evenings. I have always been one of those people who doesn't like to take pills even for a headache. But this week, I was diligent in making sure I was ingesting pain medication every four hours to try to lessen the aches in my back. On Tuesday evening, against Shawn's objections, I lined the floor with sparkly bows and wrapping paper in shades of gold and silver. Silent Night echoed throughout the house from my holiday playlist. This song and this task always reminded me of my grandmother. Bubba was a plump woman who loved to sing carols and hymns to the rooftops without a care in the world who was watching. She had bleach blonde hair that was plastered with so much hair spray it was impossible to have a single strand out of place, keeping it that way by wrapping it in toilet paper before she went to bed. Her blue eyeshadow and bright pink lipstick were applied perfectly and she always smelled like coffee and fresh laundry soap. She would decorate every single nook and cranny of her house for the holiday, from the bedsheets to the toilet cover. This is the time of year she adored most, the month we lost her and the season I always feel closest to her. Christmas was the following week and I had been stressing over finishing wrapping all of the presents.   I was annoyed and frustrated. I had a long list of tasks that I wanted to accomplish before December twenty-fifth and I was being hindered from finishing them. I quickly learned that what I had set out to do this evening was not going to happen. My back pain grew worse and I slid back into bed. I barely slept that night. The stabbing sharp jabs shot through my body followed by muscle spasms that, at some occurrences, I wasn't sure if they would ever end. I couldn't walk on my own. Shawn had to carry me to the bathroom throughout the night. As an annoying sister obviously would, I had been asking my brother, the medical professional, in the proceeding days if my symptoms were normal. By the next daybreak, he suggested I go to the urgent care. Later Wednesday morning, Shawn and I headed over to see the doctor. She performed a physical evaluation and sent me to the back to do an x-ray. I had to lay down, flat on my back, on a hard, sterile board. The pain radiated throughout my body as I closed my eyes to power through the imaging. Afterward, the doctor informed me there was nothing wrong with my back, therefore, it must be muscular. I received a shot of Toradol, a pain reliever, and a prescription for Flexeril, a muscle relaxer. She assured me that I should be feeling better within the hour. After five excruciating hours had passed, I called the doctor to advise her that I was still in the same amount of pain, if not worse, than before my visit. This conversation resulted in trying prescription lidocaine patches for the pain, which like the other medications, failed to decrease any amount of my suffering.

I was trying hard to hide the pain. It was becoming increasingly clear that something was wrong but at the same time the x-ray showed that my back was fine. Caleb was home from college for Christmas break which made my heart so overjoyed. I had missed him beyond words. Our home felt complete again now that he was back in his room while the sound of his guitar echoed through the house. I did not want him to worry about me.

I was so exhausted that I finally drifted off to sleep at some point during the night. Shawn had grown increasingly worried and had stayed up to watch me sleep, just in case I needed him. There are so many reasons I love this man and this is just one example. Shawn, who I affectionally refer to as *Muffin* on occasion, is a full-blown alpha male with the soft side that, for a long time, only I was allowed to see. My husband laughs at his own jokes, has the best belly laugh that makes everyone giggle and loves me more than anything in this whole world. I still catch him eyeing me from across the room filled with nothing but pure love.

Around 4:00 a.m. early Thursday morning, December 19, 2018, Shawn tried to help me out of bed to the bathroom. As I attempted to get up, I buckled into his arms. The sensation of pain that just ran through my body was far worse than anything I had ever experienced. It felt as if a knife had been jabbed in my spine radiating throughout my entire body. I screamed. I wailed in pain. The time had come where it was necessary to go to the emergency room but I was unable to move. Shawn wanted to call the ambulance but I did not want my child to have to witness his mother being wheeled out of the house in a stretcher. We told him we were going to the hospital for my back, assured him that I would be okay and to go back to sleep. Through screams and agony, my husband carried me to the car and we drove the ten minutes to the hospital in silence, his strong, warm hand in mine.

I was put in a cubicle in the emergency room right away. For someone who rarely takes a Tylenol, I was greatly annoyed at the medical staff who, at first, were not taking my pain seriously. I understand that there are many people who have an addiction they are unable to control and try various avenues to feed said addiction. It is a terrifying problem in this country right now. However, I was not one of them, but I was treated as if I was just there for pain pills. Finally, the doctor gave me an IV with more Toradol, ignoring the fact that it did nothing for me the day before, as well as Rebaxin, another muscle relaxer, while the nurse drew labs. When neither of these medications lessened my pain, I was sent back for a CT scan.

While we were waiting for the results, we called my Mom and Al. They wake up before the sun around 4:30 a.m. every day, Al to start work on the farm and Jean to get ready to start her work day. Still unsure of what to expect, I told them it was unnecessary to come to the hospital so my mom reluctantly headed to work. Shortly after our phone conversation, Al arrived to my room anyway, holding his signature black coffee from

17

McDonalds. As he took a seat in the corner of my small, sterile room, surrounded by the constant beeping of the machines, his pastor followed him in. I was confused. Why did he bring his preacher with him to pray for me? It's just a pulled muscle in my back, right? As it turns out, the pastor was already at the hospital visiting another patient and ran into Al. It was meant to be that day. I welcomed his prayers and his kind words.

The doctor came back in my room with a nurse who went straight over to my IV. He knelt down on the floor by my bed as the nurse started pushing something cold into my arm. "I'm sorry to have to tell you this but the CT scan showed you have a cancer called Multiple Myeloma accompanied with several lesions on your spine which have caused your L1 to collapse from a double compression fracture. We are going to give you Morphine to help with your pain now". As I lay there lost, confused, trying to make sense of what I was just told, I felt it. I could feel the cool of the Morphine streaming throughout every part of my body. Within minutes my pain was gone. I had never heard of Multiple Myeloma so I had no idea what my prognosis meant. Taking in the relief that I was finally feeling after days of being miserable, I looked down at the doctor, who was still kneeling on the floor beside my bed, and asked him if there was a cure. He informed me that, while there was not a cure to date, most of the time it was fairly treatable. My response was simple: "Fix my back and we can deal with the cancer later". And then, much to everyone's dismay, the nurse recited a story of a woman who used to work there at the desk who also had the same cancer a couple of years ago. We were expecting the follow up to be "and she is doing great" or something positive along those lines. The outcome: she didn't make it. I am not sure what would make her believe that was a good thing to share with someone who had just been diagnosed with cancer ten minutes ago but it left all our minds racing.

Immediately, we picked up our phones and began making calls. I don't think anyone who hears their phones ringing before the sun comes up is expecting good news. My heart couldn't find the words to tell my mom so Shawn took that call while I dialed my brother's number. Chad worked and lived in Columbus, where there was a greater opportunity for more advanced medical care than my hometown. I am confident that was a call that he never expected to receive. As soon as I heard his voice, I broke. Tears started trickling down my cheeks as I attempted to relay all I had just been told then slowly releasing the phone to Shawn to take over. "They are saying your sister is riddled with cancer and will need to start chemo and radiation immediately" he began. My brother had his doubts, and believing my diagnosis was wrong, demanded that we head up to Columbus right away. The ER doctor did not agree with that decision, which led to some push back from him in a failed attempt to keep me there. While I was laying there processing everything in my head, I glanced at Al sitting quietly in the corner. He was diagnosed with Squamous Cell Carcinoma cancer and went through treatment over a decade ago. I can't imagine what was going through his head knowing I would now have to go through treatments that he knew well and wouldn't wish on anyone, let alone someone he considered his daughter. He kept asking me if I needed anything or what he could do for me while trying to portray a pillar of positivity.

As a mother myself, I can't even begin to contemplate the heart break when my mom answered her phone that morning, listening to my husband relay all of the information we had just learned. He tried to reassure her that neither he nor Chad believed it was the correct diagnosis and we would find out more when additional tests were completed. She hung up the phone, dumbfounded, scared, breaking down to a gut-wrenching cry. Over a decade ago, she had been Al's caregiver during his cancer journey and she knew what all it entailed. She did not want her daughter to go through that kind of torture.

It wasn't long before I was pushed out in a wheelchair to our vehicle. Before I was discharged, we were informed that the Morphine would be wearing off soon so I was provided a couple Vicodin pills to hold me over on the two hour drive to Columbus. Unsure of how long I would be up there, we thought it was the best decision to stop at home to pack a bag. As our car slowed to a stop in our gravel driveway, I realized I had to go to the bathroom. Shawn attempted to pick me up to carry me to the house, however, by this point the Morphine had worn off completely and with every move I was screaming in pain. He put me back down and ran in to the house returning with a red solo cup. I objected immediately to his solution but quickly realized there was no other option. Through tears of embarrassment and pain, I slowly relieved myself into the plastic cup that my husband was holding in between my legs with one hand while holding me up with the rest of his body. He kept reassuring me that I was being ridiculous, but I was mortified. After quickly throwing a few clothes and toiletries in to a duffle bag, along with a soft fleece blanket for me, Shawn explained to Caleb that we were going to Columbus in order for me to have back surgery and it was okay that he return to sleep. We would touch base with him later on in the day when we had more information.

We left our quaint little home, complete with a white picket fence surrounded by lush green grass, tall trees and flowing creeks and headed north, still full of shock, questions and uncertainty.

3

Riverside

The drive to Columbus is still a blur to me. So many emotions were twirling through my head and I was graveling with immense pain again. The pills I had been given for the ride up were of little relief, if any at all. In true form, Shawn kept reassuring me that we were in this together, no matter what happens, but also was convinced that the ER doctor was wrong. Up to this point, I was a healthy young woman with very few pains or other medical issues. Two hours later, I was being wheeled into Riverside Methodist Hospital where my brother was waiting for me. Chad, who affectionately calls me "Sissy", stood a towering six feet three inches, holding a stuffed puppy and a helium smiley face balloon adorned with a Santa hat. There was never a doubt to anyone that we were siblings because our facial characteristics are one in the same, although Chad, my younger brother, was now turning grey. My eyes were a darker green, whereas his were more of a softer blue green, which he always insisted where the prettiest.

A whirlwind of tests and imaging had begun. Nurses were constantly poking my veins to draw more blood. The first doctor I saw at Riverside gave us hope. Multiple Myeloma is a blood cancer that was most commonly found in men over the age of sixty-five predominantly of African American descent. Almost all patients are anemic. Here I was the anomaly: a thirty-seven year old white woman who showed no signs of this cancer other than elevated white blood count and what appeared to be lesions on my spine. There was also concern that my kidneys were failing but, at first, there was uncertainty if it was due to my illness or from the Toradol that I received from both the urgent care as well as the emergency room. The doctor had dark brown hair and a soft smile. She assured me that, in her opinion, she was ninety percent certain that I had non-cancerous tumors formed from excess blood vessels called Hemangiomas. On the other side, my Oncologist believed that most likely it was Multiple Myeloma but that it could possibly be a cancer more or less severe. He advised me to stay calm as there were so many unanswered questions until all the test results had been reviewed. As my extensive medical team scrambled for answers, I was still struggling in agony. Pain medications were constantly being pushed through my veins or administered in a clear plastic cup. Oxycodone & Dilaudid were my narcotics and Flexeril was given to relax my back muscles that would convulse in such spasms that I would scream in pain. I couldn't get out of bed or eat anything as the pain brought on intense nausea. All we could do was wait.

We always joke that my husband has the mind of an elephant. His brain retains anything and everything he has ever read or experienced. Shawn was determined that he was not leaving this hospital as long as it was my new home. Therefore, he created a makeshift, most uncomfortable, bed on the plastic leather couch and dove right in to researching all he could find on this cancer. The studies, the treatments, the outcomes and life expectancy. Initially, what he found was that this cancer was complicated. No two cases were alike. Since all cases seemed to be different, some patients had better outcomes than others.

Multiple myeloma is typically characterized by the neoplastic proliferation of plasma cells that produce a monoclonal immunoglobulin. Put another way, Multiple Myeloma is a type of cancer that affects certain cells in your blood called plasma cells, a type of white blood cell, which are important because they produce antibodies that help fight infections in your body. These cells are created in the center of your bones, in a part called the bone marrow, where cancerous cells push out the healthy cells. In Multiple Myeloma, these plasma cells grow out of control and produce abnormal proteins called monoclonal proteins or M-proteins. This abnormal protein can build up in different parts of your body, including your bones, causing them to become weak and brittle. This may result in extensive skeletal destruction with osteolytic lesions and pathological fractures. Other side effects of having the disease in general are pain, fatigue, nausea, vomiting, diarrhea, numbness and tingling in the arms and legs, weakness, and weight loss. More serious issues can include anemia, reduced kidney function and frequent infections. And that is all prior to even starting chemotherapy.

Shawn did not sleep that first night in the hospital. I was in unbearable pain that the doctors were having a hard time getting under control. Pain medications are great, but they don't last long and patients can only have them every so often. During the early morning hours, tears poured down my cheeks from burning red eyes. I begged him over and over to make the pain go away. He would later tell me that it was so gut wrenching to him as if he were watching someone being tortured when he couldn't make it better for me. This nightmare will forever be burned in his memories. It will be something he will never forget. The next morning when the doctors made their rounds, Shawn strongly expressed his displeasure with how they were handling my uncontrollable pain. I would have relief for an hour, but the next few hours between the medicines wearing off and receiving my next dose, I was in complete agony. Eventually, the doctors changed my regimen to be given more frequently. My pain was more controlled though constantly reminding me that it was indeed still present. The increase in drugs filling my small framed body, unaccustomed to ingesting so many medications, quickly overtook my mind. For the next several days, I would disappear into a drug induced departure from reality, sleeping away this nightmare.

Enter the pee pickle. Because I was unable to get out of bed, I was offered a new device that the hospital had just recently started using. It was an external female catheter called a Purewick that resembled a giant tampon. I was advised to place it in between my legs and release myself onto it. "No way" I exclaimed. I was positive I would urinate all over the bed. After being assured over and over that this would not happen, I gave in. Anything was better than my other two options: having an internal catheter inserted in me or making it to the bathroom, which was impossible at this point. After trying it for the first time, I thought it was the best thing ever invented and I made sure to let everyone know it. I quickly named it my "pee pickle". In my drug induced excitement, every time I had to relieve myself, I would tell everyone to stop talking and pay attention. I would pee into the oversized banana shaped piece of cotton which would then flow up a tube into a canister on a pole above me beside my bed while gurgling like a pot of coffee brewing. I have always been easily amused and this whole process made me giggle with delight every single time. I can't say my family enjoyed the process as much as I did. Eventually, the Purewick became available to purchase for residential use through infomercials on tv. To this day, every time I see said commercial, I take a picture or video and forward it on to my family with a smile. My stay in Riverside was not a pleasant experience for anyone but my pee pickle was the one topic that makes us all look back and laugh. I had also found enjoyment in the smiley face Santa balloon that Chad had brought me the first day I arrived. At some point, someone thought it was a brilliant idea to tie it to the end of my bed. I spent countless hours enjoying lengthy conversations with the smiling face floating in the air in front of me.

4

Family

Two years prior to my diagnosis, we welcomed a new puppy. After recently losing our family dog, we had made the decision, as Caleb was getting ready to go to college and we were hoping to travel more, that a new dog was not in our future. However, after a tragic event that crushed my son's heart, I was left uncertain of how to mend it. In a rash decision, we brought home a tiny, playful, energetic six pound little boy. The mother in me wanted to do anything and everything that I could possibly think of to help my son through his pain. Our new puppy was a caramel colored Cavapoo with tiny white patches on his forehead and chest with soft curls and floppy ears. He had chocolate human eyes, a button nose and the sweetest round face with fur on either side that almost resembled a mustache. If you didn't know better, you would swear he was a teddy bear. I will never forget the day that Caleb came home from school, tossed his backpack on the floor and scooped up our new furry little ball into his arms. That smile and those dimples that I love so much spread over my son's face again. We named our new puppy Joey.

Joey was spoiled right from the start. We had settled on crate training him as we had other obligations during the day. That lasted all of fifteen minutes when I decided I could no longer take his whimpers. From then on out, he would wait for us to come home in the window, cuddle with us on the couch and snuggle up in one of our beds to go to sleep. Caleb loved our new pup, but between school, work, recording music and hanging out with his friends, he wasn't home often and it became clear that Joey had picked me to be his person.

Megan is my best friend. She has long flowing dark brown hair and beautiful pale green eyes with the most adorable squint when she smiles. She is often terrible at responding to text messages but will always show up to be there for me or anyone else at the drop of a dime. My mother was tasked with calling Megan to give her the news and to ask her if she would take Joey so that my family was able to go back and forth to the hospital. My friend was on her way to the post office to drop off some mail. After agreeing to pick up Joey, she hung up the phone and found a parking space. As she sat silent for a moment, trying to come to terms with what she had just been told, her emotions took over. In that parking lot she released everything that she was feeling inside. In her words, she ugly cried for what seemed like hours. Passersby scurried by her car unsure of what to think of the distraught woman inside.

Later that day, Jean, Al and Caleb started the journey to the unknown which lied two hours north. I had made it clear to everyone that I did not want Caleb to know of the possibility that I may have cancer. My diagnosis was not confidently confirmed and if and when that time came, I wanted him to hear it from me. If the doctors were wrong,

I did not want to inflict any unwarranted worry on him. He was told that I was having back surgery.

They drove the two hours to and from Columbus every day. Caleb insisted that he decorate my room for Christmas since it had become clear we would no longer be celebrating the day at home. Jean gathered a few strands of garland while he began removing ornaments from our tree. My mom suggested they take some of the decorations that were still in the box in case they were to break. Caleb insisted that the ones on the tree were my favorite, therefore, I should have those in my room. Glistening bulbs now hung from garland on my ceiling so that I could feel the holiday spirit. Cards and flowers filled the room from friends and family. Knowing how much I love all my photos, my mom taped family pictures around my temporary new home.

I was naïve to think that my son would not be aware of the rumblings of my cancer diagnosis from all of those around him as well as the medical staff shuffling in and out of my room. Looking back, I wonder what went through his head each night he came home to sleep in our empty house processing all of the unknowns we all now had to endure. Mothers are supposed to shield their children and I was the cause of his new uncertainties. My mom focused on me the best way she could think of at that time, taking care of her baby girl. She would use a shower cap prefilled with shampoo to wash my hair every other night, brush it, then braid it to keep it out of my eyes.

Chad and his wife, Paula, who was quite a bit shorter than my towering brother and had long, black hair and caramel skin, visited regularly, along with many other family and friends including my dad, Doug. He is tall, stubborn, with snow white hair and brown eyes. My current situation devastated him. I am also blessed to have an extended family from Al's side, some of which would visit me regularly, offering well wishes. As the news traveled, I began receiving nonstop text messages, many of which went unanswered due to my state of mind.

Shawn broke away to the hallway to contact work to inform them he needed some time off. It was also time for him to break down and call his parents. From the moment I met them early on when we first started dating, I fell in love with them. Bruce, his dad, is tall with tanned skin and a sense of humor he obviously passed down to his son. His mom, Carol, is a petite woman with short, sandy hair, who was also humorous with a beautiful smile. I instantly clicked with her right from the start. Neither look their age, most likely due to their continuance to play tennis several times a week. I find happiness in the little things in life and I adore the way they smell, a mix of the beach air and laundry soap. I always inhale their relaxing scent in and smile every time I see them. Shawn's parents moved to South Carolina several years ago so we don't see them as often as we would like, but I admire their love and relationship after all of these years. Being a child of divorce myself and also having gone through one of my own, I hope that Shawn and I will continue to get inspiration from his parents. Leaning up against the wall as he made this phone call, he slowly sloped down onto the floor, tears finally releasing down his face when he heard his mom's voice. Without a second thought, his parents offered to drive the ten hours it would take them to get to Columbus. Shawn assured them that it wasn't necessary at this time as we were so unsure what the future held and how long we would be there. He promised to keep them updated and advise them of any way they could be of help.

I am blessed to have so many people in my life who love me so dearly. Because of that, my heart hurts thinking back on what it was like for them to sit back with brave faces for me while breaking inside from all the unanswered questions and my future uncertainty.

5

Answers

The next day we were informed that my bones had become a nesting place for the lytic lesions that had now consumed my body. They had taken over my spine, which had caused it to collapse, as well as my ribs, my hips and my collarbone. A lytic lesion is a bone lesion resulting from cancerous plasma cells that build up in your bone marrow. My doctors were unsure if my spine was too brittle to do surgery because of this damage. When it was finally decided that a back surgery would be attempted, I spiked a fever that refused to go down. I was also having breathing issues at the time and had to be put on oxygen. Because of this, they decided to hold off on the surgery. This would happen twice more over the coming days. I would be scheduled then spike a fever. Therefore, I would continue to suffer through my pain, though somewhat controlled in my drug induced state of mind.

Shortly after learning this information, the first physician I had encountered here, who assured me that it wasn't cancer, slowly entered my room, head facing the ground. She presented me with a small single Christmas cactus with a deep red bloom. She was holding back tears as she apologized, her face riddled with guilt. She now believed that her initial assumption was wrong. At that time the nurses came in to take me down for my MRI. The doctor accompanied me downstairs to a room that I would be held in until the imaging machine was ready. She sat beside me, holding my hand in silence, until the radiology technician wheeled me away. In her mind she had failed me.

I would also need a bone marrow biopsy to confirm my suspected diagnosis. The procedure involves a large needle inserted into my hip bone where a sample of my bone marrow is collected. Luckily, I have no recollection of this painful event. We were warned that the results of the biopsy would take several days especially due to the holidays.

There are several different variants of Multiple Myeloma. My blood work showed that it was believed that I had a type known as IGG Kappa Light Chain which was the most common combination. Immunoglobulins, aka antibodies, are proteins that your body uses to fight off infections. There are five types of immunoglobulins, each with two heavy proteins paired together with two light chains. Myeloma cells produce abnormal immunoglobulins called monoclonal proteins or M-Spike which are unable to fight infections. One of the reasons it was so hard to diagnose for me was because I have a rare kind known as Non-Secretory, which means I do not have the M-spike. Multiple Myeloma is only found in less than five percent of patients under the age of forty. Only three percent of all myeloma patients have Non-Secretory. Here I reside in the very rare percentage of both. Due to this rarity, I was asked to sign paperwork to allow future medical teams to learn from my diagnosis. The normal range for the kappa light chains is between 3.3 – 19.4. Mine was 4024.0.

December 23, 2018: my back surgery was finally going to happen. My mom was determined to see me before I went into surgery that morning. It was a last minute decision that left Jean, Al and Caleb rushing to arrive to the hospital that day. In doing so, they got lost and time was ticking down. I would soon be leaving for the operation room. My mom kept calling Shawn, begging him to stall them in any way possible. Running through the sterile hospital hallways, then charging out of the elevator, my mom rushed to the side of the gurney just as I had exited my room. Holding back tears, full of fear and faith, she kissed me on my forehead and made sure I knew just how much she loved me as I started to drift off. I, of course, have always known how lucky I am that God chose her to be my mother and I have never doubted her unwavering love for me. I cannot imagine how it felt that day for her standing alone in a scarce hallway watching her baby girl disappear into the elevator. All anyone left in my room could do now was sit and wait until my surgery was complete and pray that it was successful enough to relieve the absorbent amount of pain that they have had to stand by and watch me endure the last several days.

I remember lying on a freezing cold hard metal surface surrounded by glaring bright lights. In an instant, I was counting backwards to drift off to sleep. My surgery was successful, and much to my surprise, the incision was so minuscule that we questioned whether or not I had actually had surgery. Unsure if my brittle bones could support a fusion at this time, it was determined I would have a vertebroplasty, which was a quick fix, filling in the gap with cement. The intense stabbing pain had lessened immediately. Although the surgery was a success, the toll the damage had done on my body still remained. I was still unable to walk and I was now wrestling with a different kind of pain. I would have a long road to recovery. But as I had said to the ER doctor that first night, my back was on the road to recovery so it was time for me to focus on my cancer.

6

Christmas

Instead of our family sitting around our Christmas tree adorned with heirloom ornaments, glittered gold bulbs and twinkling lights, we were all packed into a tiny hospital room. Our home would sit empty without all the familiar aromas of holiday dinner simmering on the stove and pecan tarts baking in the oven. I was still unable to walk so I had to be escorted downstairs in my wheelchair to the cafeteria for our Christmas dinner. A free holiday medley was being offered to celebrate the occasion. This would be the first time I had eaten anything since I had arrived here. A small plate of french fries would be my holiday meal this year. As I sat at the end of the table, I watched my family as they consumed their cafeteria feast. They had all given up their traditional holiday routine to sit around a sterile table in the basement of a hospital indulging in mediocre food. Although I knew my life would never be the same again, I took in this moment to be thankful of just how lucky I am to have these people in my life.

We had decided to exchange most of our gifts whenever the time came that I would return home. Jean had brought Caleb his presents overflowing in a dark green Santa sack with his name across the front in red and silver glitter. Since Chad and Paula lived in Columbus and were unsure when they would be able to make it back down to Marietta, we opened some of their gifts as well. The best gift that day: my brother announced that I was going to be an aunt! They had been trying for several years to get pregnant and were losing hope. In my drugged-up state of mind, I had related my situation and their news somehow to a movie I had seen. I started crying, reciting that I was going to die so that their baby could have my soul to live. Obviously, it was complete nonsense that nobody knew how to react to my blubbering mess. Although they didn't blame me for my strange reaction, I apologized profusely for this embarrassment once I was told what I said a few weeks later. This child was a miracle baby and I was beyond excited to become an aunt for the first time.

When the day was coming to an end and the darkness had taken over the sky outside, Caleb slid a chair over to my bed and placed tiny earbuds into my ears. He was a talented musician and songwriter who had written me a song as he sat alone at home each night he left the hospital. As the words began to flow, my heart was full and broken at the same time. As he strummed his guitar and sang his heart out, tears slid slowly down my cheeks. I hated that he had to watch me go through this and the fear he endured with his mother's future uncertainty. The words of the song made it clear that, although we had tried to shield him for the time being, he knew I had cancer. We were still awaiting my biopsy results, but I think we were all still living in denial, praying for a miracle. I loved this song beyond words. It was special, from the heart and the talent of my child. As my mother would say: my cup runneth over. He included my birthday, along with things that only our family would understand, like when I was younger and had my own pretend newsroom known as Rainbow News. I will treasure this song for my lifetime as well as this moment frozen in time. At a time we all wished was a nightmare we would awake from, all I could see was a beautiful heartfelt memory given to me by my child who I was overwhelmingly proud of for so many reasons.

"In the Morning"

Frozen heart and a messy home
Things I left you when I found out
you had cancer of the bone
Shaky voice like a telephone
we drove our car to the red lot
There's no place to feel sorry
In the morning through the window shade
When the light pressed up against your shoulder blade
We could hear what you were thinking
All the glory that the Lord has made
The complications you could do without
the dryness of the mouth
Tuesday night at a bible study Jean will take my hand
We'll be praying for your body
I'm sure I'll see you smiling
I remember at our old house how hard you worked
While I would hang out with Papaw drawing airplanes
In the morning at the top of the stairs
when we all found out

What you knew that night
and you told me you were scared
All the glory when you run outside
with your shirt tucked in
And your shoes untied I'll have no need to follow you
Rainbow News to the Rainbow Brite
Chad will say they're so trite he will always be the favorite
Just a team made of you and Shawn
from the beach of Florida
To our front lawn in the Miller Olympics
In the morning when you finally go and the nurse runs in
With no head hung low I know we will follow you
In the morning in the window shade
It's the Third of April it's a holiday
There's no doubt I see you smiling
All the glory that the Lord has made
and the complications
When I see his face in the morning in the window
All the glory when he took our place
He took my shoulders and he shook my face
And he takes and he takes and he takes

7

Confirmation

After days of sticking my veins repetitively, they started to blow one after another. When no more blood was being extracted from my tortured veins, it was decided I would have an Ultrasound Guided Peripheral Catheter IV placed in my upper arm. My brother had previously been a trainer for this procedure so he took interest in watching the nurse begin to place it in my arm. Chad knew right away that the nurse was doing it incorrectly: botching the first attempt, followed by a multitude of mistakes that could pose a potential infection risk. Within minutes, my protective brother demanded the nurse cease the procedure and located his supervisor, who replaced said nurse, to complete the placement into my arm. We would later learn that the nurse had been fired for the unsanitary procedure he was performing on me.

I had quickly learned that I liked some nurses more than others. In particular, I had grown fond of a tall, thin nurse with long red hair, who I had named *Sansa* as she reminded me of the girl from Game of Thrones. She was kind, compassionate and great at taking my blood. Early on in one of my drug comas, I attempted to sweet talk a male nurse and bribe him with my body if he would break me out of the hospital. I am sure that my husband enjoyed watching me flirt with the young man but he just sat back and laughed at me. On the flip side, I did not like one of the nurses who was simply unable to get any blood out of my arm and would make several attempts to find viable veins in other parts of my body. The arm catheter was put in for a reason: more of a port, they could open up to extract blood when needed rather than sticking needles in me constantly. Her incompetence to figure out the arm catheter was not acceptable in my condition. At one point, Shawn had reached his breaking point with her and walked her backwards out of my room, refusing to let her take my blood, demanding a new nurse. I was surrounded by a protective force of love from my family that nobody was going to break.

The day after Christmas I started physical therapy. I was given a walker and attempted to take a few steps in the hallway. Hospital gown not fully closed in the back, bright yellow socks with rubbered bottoms and messy braided hair. It was evident that my recovery would be a long road. At thirty-seven years old, I would be using a walker or wheelchair for the foreseeable future. Although I had not been eating, I had gained eight pounds this week from the fluids being pumped throughout my body. My doctors were insistent that I try to eat something, but the only food I could tolerate was Rice Krispies cereal. The remainder of my stay, that was the only thing I would ingest.

The following evening, my oncologist visited me with the results of my biopsy. It had taken longer to process due to the holidays which had left all of us on pins and needles. The middle-aged man with buzzed soft grey hair softly went on to tell us that my bone marrow was 50-60% myeloma cancer cells. I had a Monosomy of 8, 13 and 14 and a 1q deletion. A monosomy is the absence of one member of a chromosome whereas the deletion is missing altogether. We had no idea what this information meant and would learn more down the road. My doctor advised me that he had spoken to a former colleague of his, Dr. Cawley, who practiced in Marietta and, although she was not taking new patients at this time, he had persuaded her to take me on as she was the best in the area. I was grateful.

My initial treatment would consist of three medications. Velcade (Bortezomib) is a type of therapy known as a proteasome inhibitor that works by disrupting cellular processes killing cancer cells. It would be a shot in my stomach twice a week. Dexamethasone was a high dose steroid that can stop white blood cells from traveling to areas of the body where cancerous myeloma cells are causing damage. It also decreases swelling and inflammation in those areas providing short term relief of pain and pressure. Revlimid (Lenalidomide) is an immunomodulatory drug (iMiDs) that works against cancer cells by supporting the function of the immune system. This medication would simply be one pill once a day. Through the shock, I asked if I would lose my hair. To my surprise, the answer was no. He sat with us until we could no longer come up with questions or concerns, wished us well and departed for the evening.

As the doctor stepped out of the door, Shawn leaned over the side of the bed to wrap his arms around me, his grasp so tight I could barely breathe. We both sank into each other as tears poured down our faces. It had been confirmed. I had cancer. There was no more hope or denial. This was it. It was not supposed to be this way but we had to succumb to reality. After we had begun to calm down from our emotional release, Shawn leaned back, wiped my tears away and looked me straight in my green eyes, now burning red. "You are going to fight with all you have because you are the love of my life and I need you". This moment was the most raw, emotional experience of my life. Our least favorite nurse had been standing outside my door while the doctor had been giving us the gut-wrenching news. She did not feel the need to give us time to grieve and came in to take my vitals shortly after he walked out the door. Shawn was livid, made her acutely aware of her insensitivity and kicked her out of the room accordingly. Checking my blood pressure would have to wait. After we had come to terms with the plan for the foreseeable future, we felt somewhat of a relief that at least we now had answers. We took to the task of breaking the news to our close families and friends with the understanding I wanted to tell Caleb in person.

We were given a large packet of information and papers to sign in order to administer these medications. Revlimid is a derivative of Thalidomide, which was originally used in the fifties and sixties for morning sickness in pregnant women, until it became known it caused severe birth defects. It was made abundantly clear that I could not become pregnant. In addition to the effects of the actual cancer, these medications are notorious for a host of other life-altering side effects: severe itching/rash, insomnia, swelling of the legs, anemia, fatigue, nausea, vomiting, diarrhea, asthenia, dizziness, muscle cramps and spasms, increased upper respiratory infections, and random fevers. And those are just the popular side effects. The actual list of side effects is pages long, all of which I read thoroughly. Sometimes, ignorance is bliss, but my brother jokes that I may be the only person/patient who reads every syllable of those little bible-like booklets that accompany medications. It had become clear that the next several months were going to be miserable.

Early the next morning as the sun came up, we were ecstatic to hear the news I was being discharged today. While waiting on the pharmacy to fill all of my prescriptions, I received my first shot of Velcade in my stomach. It wasn't terrible and I would rather have a quick prick in the belly than sit for hours a day for an infusion. My husband packed up all of our belongings around the room that had become our home for the last several days. My brother had encouraged him to stay at his house for a good night's sleep, or at least a hot shower, but eventually gave up once he realized Shawn would not be leaving me. He sat by my side, day after day, struggling within himself, but providing me with the strong face and comfort I needed. I am certain he was ready to crawl into our plush bed at home. After what seemed like an eternity, my paperwork was finalized and, holding a paper bag filled to the brim with orange bottles, I was loaded up in my new wheels and headed out the door to go home.

8

Home

As we pulled into our long gravel driveway, a sense of relief poured over me. I could see Joey barking and wagging his tail in our oversized front window that overlooked the hayfields. Over the last couple of days, Al had constructed a ramp so that I was able to get in the front door in my wheelchair. Jean and Al were there, eager to welcome me home. As Shawn began to help me out of the car, the cool air hit my face. Fresh air. I took it all in, unaware of just how much I had missed it over the last several days. I could hear my wind chimes bellowing in the slight breeze, one for each of my lost grandparents, Bubba and Pappy, a reminder my angels were always nearby. Joey was beaming with excitement to see us. As soon as the door opened, he rushed over with so much momentum that his little paws were sliding on the slick tile floors. He was eager to jump on us, to lick our ears and faces and receive all the love he had been longing for while we were gone. The moment he saw me, Joey halted to a stop. He knew in an instant something was wrong. Rather than pounce on me to shower me with his love, he simply placed a gentle paw on my leg. Shawn helped me out of my chair onto the sofa where a foam lumbar pillow now resided. I was required to wear a back brace: a hard, most uncomfortable girdle. Once it was wrapped around me, it conformed to my small frame, sucking my body into it. The brace and the pillow were supposed to aid in my comfort and healing. Joey waited somewhat patiently as I got situated, trying desperately to reach a level of comfort I could manage. Once a soft fleece blanket was draped across my legs, he leaped onto the couch to lay his curly head on my lap and pressed his warm fur against my body. From this point forward, he would never leave my side. If I moved, so did he. I looked around our living room to the tree twinkling in the corner and the photos adorning the walls. I closed my eyes with a sigh of relief. I was home.

Caleb sat down beside me on the couch. I took his hand in mine and forged deep inside my soul to find strength. "My biopsy came back that I do have cancer" I began. I went on to explain that I had my first dose of chemotherapy that morning. I watched his big brown eyes well up while he tried to show his strength. I hated myself for the pain I was causing him. My job as a mother was to protect him and shield him from ever hurting. I promised him that we were going to get through this nightmare and everything would be okay. As he wrapped his arms around me, I could no longer hold back my tears.

I was exhausted from the ride home. The boys transferred me over to my oversized electric recliner boasting large green and yellow flowers. I loved this chair. It had been custom made for me for my birthday one year in this spectacular print called *lemoncello*. I was forced to take a couple bites of Rice Krispies cereal over my objections. I was uncomfortable and nauseous with absolutely no desire to eat. Joey promptly took his spot on my lap with paw stretched out on my leg. I had another protector. I ingested the plethora of pills sent home with me and drifted off to sleep, sunk deep into my floral cushion.

The next day we celebrated our Christmas together. I changed out of my yoga pants and sweatshirt in to a shimmery grey sweater. I completed my ensemble with a gold and white pearl necklace. My mom had arranged all of the silver and gold glittered gifts under the tree in perfect order. Christmas carols played silently in the background. I made an attempt to eat a small amount of the holiday feast Jean had prepared. We passed around the colored boxes to each other, eager to discover what was kept inside. Caleb gifted me a stuffed elephant named *Ellie* to keep me company and gave it a home at the top of my headboard, where it still resides. For a long time, I sat stoic in my chair, back brace plastered over top of my holiday attire, staring at the tree in all its glory. My life would now become known as "before cancer" and "after cancer" and I was taking it all in. We tried to make the best of our holiday celebration under the circumstances. My family was together, and at the end of the day, that is what most.

We had been trying to get tickets to see the Hamilton Broadway play for several months. I was finally able to acquire three tickets for the show in Pittsburgh, Pennsylvania for the beginning of January. I was beaming with excitement to gift them to Caleb for Christmas.

Obviously, I would not be able to go with him now, however, I encouraged him to use the tickets to see it with friends or to take his grandparents. He rejected my offer, suggested that I sell them and we would all go together at another time. This broke my heart as I knew how badly he had been wanting to see this play. I begged him to go, but in the end, I was unsuccessful. Another thing cancer has already taken from our family.

I have always been that person who believes everything happens for a reason. After years of talking about adding an addition to our house, we had finally begun the renovations the previous year. Our old farmhouse had been updated here and there but we needed more space. Jean and I love a good project and work amazingly well together. We took it upon ourselves one weekend to paint all the kitchen cabinets a crisp shade of ivory white to compliment the grey swirled quartz countertops. The island received a fresh coat of sage green. Shawn was a master of all trades around the house and could fix just about anything. But this renovation would be massive. All new grey tile flooring, which resembled wood grain, needed to be installed throughout. Caleb's bedroom, along with the master bedroom, were to be enlarged, as well as an addition of an ensuite. The renovations were long and brutal, as we lived among construction for several weeks, but it was all completed last year. Our ensuite bathroom now consisted of a large walk-in shower with geometric tiles varying from textured white, blue sea glass and shimmery metals. I am now required to use a shower seat as well as handles suctioned to the glass in order to bathe myself. I haven't the slightest idea how I would have accomplished getting in and out of the old tub shower in our main bathroom. During the renovation, we replaced our queen bed with a king size, complete with an adjustable frame that, up to this point, had never been used. The universe knew I would need these amenities before I did. The adjustable bed allowed me to sleep upright and the new shower provided the ease of getting in and out. It was all right there together for the days I was unable to remove myself from what now seemed like my own apartment within my house. As Shawn picked me up into bed that evening, my eyes scanned the pale blue walls, the abundance of beach décor and the two recliners on either side of the bed. One for each of us. Shawn's was deep chestnut leather and mine was pale aqua covered in outlines of large white flowers. He pulled the quilt over top of me and I could feel the soft coolness of my sheets over top my plush mattress topper. I had become accustomed to the inflatable hospital beds with scratchy sheets. This was like lying on a fluffy cloud. He kissed my forehead while reassuring me we would get through this and everything would be alright. I love this man of mine.

The evening following our celebration, Caleb woke up vomiting, his face burning with a fever. In this moment, he was terrified of getting me sick in my fragile state. He called my mom, who he refers to as Mamaw, to ask if he could stay there until he recovered. My heart was in shambles. It was my job to take care of my sick child. I attempted to go to him, to hold a cool cloth on his head while he hovered over the commode but Shawn held me back. I was angry that cancer was already taking my ability to be a doting mom. Jean and Al lived next door down a gravel road in a dark cedar wood farmhouse which resided on a hundred-acre farm, complete with three barns, one of which we were married in. My mom stayed up with my son the rest of the night, holding wet washcloths on his head, as he relayed back and forth between the bed and the bathroom.

9

The First Cycle

This year, we celebrated New Year's Eve at the Strecker Cancer Center here in Marietta. It is a small, quaint building that is attached to the hospital. The center of the waiting room boasts a circular fireplace radiating heat towards every chair. Books, magazines and brochures line the shelves for patients to engage in while waiting their turn. I was greeted by a sweet lady with short blonde hair and a friendly smile sitting at the front desk. We took our seats next to a small fish tank and began perusing a pamphlet on Multiple Myeloma to pass the time. Shawn could sense that I was growing nervous and began slowly rubbing my back. A nurse opened a door to call us back to the exam room, pronouncing my name incorrectly as "Leah". Being used to this scenario, I did not correct her. Initially, my parents had planned to name me Anna Leigh, but at some point, changed it to Leigh Ann. Middle names aren't usually shown in medical or school records, therefore, I had become accustom to going with the flow when it came to my name. Most of my family refer to me as *Annie* whereas Al calls me *Leigh Annie*. I tend to write my name together as *Leighann* in a hurry and it drives my mom crazy. She scolds me by reminding me that it is not how she named me. Sometimes I do it on purpose just to get her going.

A young male nurse with strawberry blonde hair entered the room to take my blood for lab work. Chemo patients are not allowed to have their treatments if certain numbers are too low such as white blood count or neutrophils. Much to my surprise, these labs are resulted within a few minutes here. While waiting for my bloodwork to return, Dr. Cawley enters the room wearing black scrubs underneath her white coat. She is tall with a gorgeous shade of light auburn red hair that falls just below her ears. As she begins to speak, I instantly grow calmer as she exuberates compassion and kindness. Introductions are made, followed by a quick trip down memory lane as she and Shawn reminisce about playing tennis together in school. Moving the chair aside, she kneels down beside the bed I was sitting on. On her clipboard of plain white copy paper, she begins drawing pictures and bubble charts surrounded by written explanations. I immediately love her. She chose to position herself face to face with me and explain in such detail on paper to show how much she truly cares. I have always been a visual person. I need to look at things to comprehend them well. My binder of doctors' notes would also come in handy once chemo brain began. The outlook seems optimistic. I am young and otherwise healthy. My regimen will be as follows: Velcade shots in my stomach twice a week for two weeks followed by one week off. Revlimid pills every day for twenty-one days then seven days off. Dexamethasone one day a week but all ten pills at once. The week off is to give my body a little time to repair itself and raise my white blood count and neutrophils that control my immune system. If all went well, I would only need five of these cycles. The male nurse returned to administer my second shot of Velcade. The needle was in and out of me in seconds and this time I had felt its wrath. I was advised that I also needed to make an appointment with a Multiple Myeloma specialist at the James Cancer Center at the Ohio State University in Columbus. We left my appointment confident, with a better understanding of my diagnosis. Later that evening a small red bruise grew from under the bandage on my stomach.

I woke up the next morning with my ears burning and knew instantly I had a fever. Any temperature over 100.4 was an immediate call to my doctor. Even though it was New Year's Day, Dr. Cawley returned my call within seconds. The emergency room wasn't ideal for my fragile immune system but the offices were closed for the holiday. The decision was made that I would go to the hospital but she would call to advise them I was on my way. When we arrived, I was immediately pushed back to an exam room where a doctor and three nurses were waiting for me. While the doctor began his exam, one nurse extracted blood from my shriveled veins while the other two conducted other tests on me. Dr. Cawley was given their findings within twenty minutes then I was being wheeled out the sliding doors to my car. My body had been fighting a reaction to the Velcade. It was a whirlwind, but I had felt like royalty.

The following day, I had my second appointment in the chemo ward of the Cancer Center. Each patient had their own cubicle complete with a small television. Several nurses all dressed in teal, my favorite color, scurried between their assigned patients for the day. A tall, elderly man wearing a dark blue volunteer vest offered me a cup of chili. My appetite was still lost, which meant I was still living on my cereal. When I politely passed on his offer, he encouraged me to take the crackers at the very least. I obliged but did not finish them. My veins had become so busted that retrieving anything from them had become complicated and painful. After another prick in the stomach for the Velcade we were able to go home. Within a couple of hours my temperature would spike again. My mother had made the decision early on that she would practically move in with us. She would arrive to our house immediately after work and go to her home only to sleep. We spent the day attempting to maintain my fever with Tylenol and my mother. Hours went by where she alternated placing a cold cloth on my head and replenishing it with dunking it in the ice bath beside my bed. Her heart tried to maintain strength but the parent in her was riddled with concern though she put on a brave face. My husband did not sleep that night. He laid in bed watching me sleep, waking me up every hour for a temperature check as well as a Tylenol dose when the time warranted.

A few days later, I would begin taking the high dose steroid, Dexamethasone, ten pills all at once. I was hopeful that it would give me some of the strength and energy I had been lacking the last few weeks. I was warned that these pills would keep me up at night, however, I did not realize I would be awake for a couple of days, followed by a hard crash coming down off it. I grew to have a love / hate relationship with these pills. During my up time, I was dead set on finishing my annual digital scrapbook album. I have always had a deep love for photography and looked forward to finalizing my album the beginning of every January. My mom insisted that I don't stress about finishing it so soon. In the back of my head, I knew that if something happened to me, I needed the album to be completed. When the hard bound smell of freshly printed paper plastered with my favorite photographs arrived in the mail a few weeks later, I was content.

The final day of my first cycle came quickly. A couple of the nurses complimented me on how much better I looked. Although nice words are always good to hear, this made me wonder just how terrible did I appear the last two weeks? "You look so much healthier today" one nurse smiled. My fourth Velcade finally resulted in no fever! My body had grown accustomed to its wrath. The nurses challenged me to be out of my wheelchair by my next appointment. The Cancer Center had become like another home where the medical staff who resided there were quickly becoming my second family.

I was progressing well in my lab results so it was suggested to me that I would officially only need five

cycles of my regimen. I do much better in life with a plan.
Now I had one. My first cycle down. Four more to go.

10

In Between

All of the chemicals that have been ravaging inside my body the last couple of weeks finally caught up with me. It has grown difficult to even stay awake. I have been sleeping away the majority of my days this week. It has been frustrating for me to feel so incompetent. I started physical therapy and have been learning to navigate my home with a walker. Joey has maintained his spot next to me in whatever I do. My trainer is amazed by his attachment to my side, guiding me along my walker, as I travel up and down my hallways learning to walk again. I am never without my protective puppy by my side. The last few weeks I have spent masking my pain with narcotics and muscle relaxers. The stubbornness in me tries to suffer as long as I can take it before succumbing to the pills.

A gift from my brother arrived in the mail today. When I open it, I find it overflowing with rubber burgundy bracelets that read *LouStrong* on one side and Multiple Myeloma on the other. Burgundy is the cancer ribbon color for Multiple Myeloma. Chad tells me that *Leigh Ann Strong* was too long, *Annie Strong* didn't seem to sound right so he settled on *LouStrong*. Lou was a nickname given to me by friends I used to work with at a restaurant. It started out as Lulubelle but at some point, was shortened to simply Lou. Shawn has always called me Lou, as well as friends with whom I worked with back in the day. I had started a blog on Facebook to update my friends and family who had been constantly checking in on me. I had become so tired and unable to respond to everyone individually and this had allowed me to share my journey with my concerned loved ones. It is also a platform for my tribe to send me notes wishing me well, full of prayers and positivity. Sometimes, those comments were all it took to brighten my day. I immediately posted a picture of the bracelets which resulted in everyone requesting one of their own. I was being supported further by those walking around town with the burgundy bands around their wrists.

I had become very accustomed to having my son back home again these last several weeks over his holiday break. The time had come for him to return to college. Ignoring my objections, he had made the decision to continue to return home every Thursday evening then drive back to school on Sunday nights. I assured him repeatedly that I would be fine and that I wanted him to spend the remainder of his first year of college enjoying his weekends there. My pleas fell on deaf ears. While my heart was always overjoyed to have him home, I held so much guilt that his first year of college would be remembered in this way.

A schedule to babysit me was decided on. Since Al was retired from his full-time job, he would take on the appointments as well as all other times Shawn and Jean were at work. My mom would arrive after work until it was time for her to catch up on rest of her own. Shawn was home every evening so it wasn't necessary for her to give up her life to be with me every free moment she had. Though to her, a mother's job is never done.

Immediately following my arrival home, a meal train had been set up between my friends and family. Every night a new dinner would be left at my doorstep, usually complete with a dessert. Boxes of Rice Krispies, along with variants featuring chocolate or other new flavors, would usually accompany the dinners in case cereal was still all I could stomach that evening. Shawn's mom mailed a care package that included a Willow Tree figurine as well as a double batch of her famous chocolate chip cookies. Her recipe includes walnuts, which I don't care for in my baked goods, so she has always made me my own batch without them. I started receiving gifts of blankets, robes, coloring books and religious books of hope. It was humbling to watch everyone rally around me. I received cards and messages from friends I had not seen in years other than a random Facebook post from time to time. It is comforting to know how many people love and support you over the years.

I was advised early on that my chemo regimen would greatly reduce my immune system. I would have to take steps to try to protect myself from getting sick in order to shield me from the possibility I may end up in the hospital. I was wearing masks for cancer before the whole world would wear them for the COVID pandemic. My husband, my constant protector, placed an oversized bottle of hand sanitizer outside our front door. For the very few people who were deemed allowed inside my house, after passing his questionnaire, they were required to douse themselves in the germ-killing serum. Because of this, Shawn quickly earned himself the name "The Warden" and wore it proudly.

My estate work had obviously grown very far behind. I was unable to go to the office given my weak immune system. My boss was kind enough to set up a program that would allow me to log in to my work computer from my laptop at home. I felt guilty that I was only able to do a minuscule amount of work due to my constant pain and fatigue. On the flip side, I was also excited to do something that seemed somewhat normal even if it were only for a small amount of time. Some days, I wasn't able to do anything but sleep. My boss has always been sympathetic, supportive and understanding throughout my journey. I will always be eternally grateful for how he handled my diagnosis. Eventually, I would have to discontinue my work life when it became too much for me to handle.

I had been holding on to hope that I would be able to go to the upcoming concerts we had planned to attend, knowing it was impossible. We held tickets to see three country music artists over the next couple of months: Justin Moore, Jon Pardi and Garth Brooks. It pained me to finally list them all for sale on social media. We were lucky to have a VIP package allowing us to meet Jon Pardi prior to the concert. I emailed his team explaining my situation, then providing them with the names of my friends who would now be meeting him instead. A few days after reading a very sweet reply, boasting an encouraging "we hope to see you at a show once you are better", they sent me a surprise black bomber jacket with my name embroidered in white on the front and a large bright blue and orange Jon Pardi logo on the back. A note was included wishing me a quick recovery with the hope this gift would brighten my spirits. The fact that a famous music artist took the time to care so much about my predicament made me like him even more.

On top of everything else I was dealing with, I had to add the constant phone calls to grants and insurance at the top of my list. There is nothing more exhausting than spending hours on the phone dealing with insurance. You pay the premium which should mean everything should automatically be taken care of, right? I would quickly learn this was not the case. Claims were processed incorrectly or not at all, requiring yet another call usually resulting in being transferred to another representative. I had managed to meet my max out of pocket for both last year and this year in a matter of two weeks. Surgeries and chemotherapy are ridiculously expensive. My Revlimid alone was more than $28,000.00 every month before insurance contributed. My medical bills were starting to pile up. It was all beginning to be overwhelming. A friend of mine suggested a fundraiser to lessen my financial burden. My brother designed a pale grey t-shirt that read *LouStrong* below a burgundy butterfly with a cancer ribbon between the wings for the front. The back was covered with an abundance of burgundy butterflies varying in shapes and sizes scattered overtop the phrase "No one fights alone". Family, friends and acquaintances, as well as people I had never met before, were all wearing my shirts in solidarity. They raved about, not only the design, but also the softness of the shirts which felt like silk against the skin.

I opened my phone to a Facebook message from the nurse practitioner who had initially examined me at the urgent care. She inquired if I minded her reaching out on social media, noting that I had been on her mind. She had called me while I was at Riverside as a follow up to my visit to see how I was doing. My reply had been "Well, I'm in the hospital with a broken back and cancer so I've been better" followed by a giggle. Even though she had apologized for her failure that day, it was evident that she was holding on to guilt. I am not sure how a collapsed spine is overlooked on an x-ray but I held nothing against her. She was a cute, young woman with long blonde hair. She appeared new to her role and everyone makes mistakes.

My first week off my regimen flew by but it was time to begin my next cycle.

11

The Second Cycle

I woke up the day before my second cycle was to begin unable to get out of bed. My entire body ached more so than the usual as I pushed myself too hard the day before during physical therapy. Being bedridden all day resulted in a complete emotional breakdown. I was frustrated with the progress my body was making and learning to walk again, with all the rules and restrictions that I now had to uphold, as well as all the cancer had taken from me so far. When I first arrived home, I was so weak that Shawn would have to hold me in the shower, water flowing down over the two of us and lather me with soap. Since then, I have progressed by being able to use my shower chair but still require assistance in getting in and out after washing myself. My husband still has to help me put my clothes on every day as well as guide me to the bathroom. Today, due to a mix of my stubbornness and will to do things on my own, I attempted to head to the bathroom by myself via my walker but soon found myself laying on the cold tile floor. I had tripped over the scale. Shawn bolted down the hallway and embraced me into his strong arms simultaneously examining me to make sure I had not injured myself further. My tears waterfalled down my face as I released everything I had been feeling, my head buried in his chest soaking his navy blue shirt. He echoed again and again "I'm right here honey" and "I got you baby". After what seemed like hours, but I'm confident were mere minutes, he scooped me up into his arms, tucked me in bed and told me to get some rest, followed by a kiss on my forehead. I needed this man so much and he had to leave me for a couple of days overnight for a work meeting he was required to attend. I had constantly reassured him that I would be fine, however, inside I was terrified of being without him.

I had also been trying to hide my fear of starting the Revlimid the next day. I was unable to take it during my first cycle due to the insurance process trying to get them to approve covering part of it. Every month, in order to receive my chemo, I would have to go through a series of questions, referred to as a survey, asking me if I had donated blood, missed any dosage or thought that I may be pregnant. I also had to divulge whether or not I had had intercourse with a male partner, and if so, what two forms of birth control I used given the severity of the birth defects this medication could cause. Following the survey, I would have to listen to a pharmacist recite a novel from her computer explaining to me all of the side effects I may experience as well as all of the many things I should not do while taking the Revlimid. I would have to do this over and over again every single month even if I myself had memorized the words.

The Revlimid comes packaged in a bright yellow bag and reads "CAUTION: CHEMOTHERAPY DRUG OBSERVE SAFETY PRECAUTIONS FOR HANDLING". The enclosed pamphlet lists a surplus of the most common side effects including diarrhea, nausea, chemo rash, itching, swelling, fatigue, tiredness, weakness, insomnia, muscle cramps, joint aches, shaking, pain as well as cold or flu symptoms. The more severe outcomes include birth defects, liver failure, risk of developing new cancers and increased risk of death. Several of the warning paragraphs began with "a very bad and sometimes deadly reaction" as well as "It can cause very bad health problems that may not go away, and sometimes death". I feel like whomever was responsible for choosing the wording for this brochure could have chosen a better description other than "very bad". My anxiety heightened as I scanned over the black and white print.

The next morning, Al and I headed to the hospital for my first pet scan. I was escorted into a small dark closet with only one chair. After pushing a radiation serum through my IV and being warned that I would be radioactive for forty-eight hours so I shouldn't go around pregnant women or children, I was told to sit back and relax why the chemicals moved throughout my body. Al was not allowed to accompany me in the room since they wanted me to have no disturbances. An hour later, I would pass him sitting in the hallway on a hard wooden chair where he would assure me that's where he would be when I was finished. I have always been claustrophobic so I have never been a fan of being stuck in a tube to complete a test. Today, radiology technician offered me a face mask to place over my eyes. This lady changed my life. While

I still don't enjoy imaging tests through a tunnel, the eye mask allowed me to relax without the fear of opening my eyes to see that I am only an inch away from the top of the cylinder. On the way home, we stopped by the store to get a few groceries. Donning my mask and walker, I was eager to peruse the aisles making sure to put a package of Oreos and toasted ravioli, both favorites of my mother, into the cart for my girls' night with her that evening. It was the first time I was able to go anywhere other than appointments for the last three weeks.

Shawn was having a really hard time being away from me, knowing it was the first test to date that he had not been able to attend with me. That afternoon, Megan came over to babysit me since Jean and Al had a couple of things they needed to take care of for a while. I was so excited to be able to spend time with her, making girl talk, crying about my diagnosis and for the first time, being able to express real emotions about my cancer. The role for my husband and my parents is to encourage me that everything is going to be okay. A best friend's role is to support me but also to tell me it's alright that it sucks and it's not fair. I need both of these things in my life in order to achieve balance. We spent the afternoon reminiscing of good times, being upset over my ordeal, as well as alternating laughs and tears. She told me the story of waking up to my furry pup staring at her in bed at three o'clock in the morning while she was watching him when I was in the hospital. Unbeknownst to her, Shawn and Joey wake up at the same time in the middle of the night to indulge in peanut butter toast. As soon as I mentioned peanut butter toast while explaining this to Megan, Joey eagerly ran over to the cabinet where we keep the peanut butter, sat down with his paw up in the air, waiting patiently for his favorite snack. We both burst out in laughter. Something so minuscule was just what my soul needed. It's the little things that make a big impact. After a long exhausting day, Jean and I indulged in fried ravioli and Oreos for dinner and enjoyed a movie together. That night, my mom and I slept side by side in my king size bed, Joey annoyed that she was there and trying his best to push her out.

When I awoke the next morning, Al was sitting quietly in the chair beside my bed just in case I needed anything. I have no idea how long he had been there and felt terrible imagining him sitting there bored for hours. I had been doing better getting around with my walker as of late so I rolled myself in to the living room. Two things I was sick of hearing: drink more water and eat more protein. Neither of which I enjoyed doing at the moment. Everything I put in to my mouth tasted like metal. I had read on a Facebook group I followed that switching to plastic silverware may help so I had made that swap a couple of days ago. If I didn't want to do something I would just get an "okay honey" from my mom, however, Al made a game out of it by hoarding my water. He was determined to get me better as quickly as possible. If I wanted a drink, he made me shuffle my walker across the room to get it, cheering me on, looking past my annoyance. But I needed this as well. Someone to push me when I did not want to put in the effort.

Later that afternoon, Al and I arrived at the Cancer Center ready for the results of my pet scan. Waiting for test results is nerve wracking. I wondered what Al was thinking, walking in to the chemo room for the first time since he went into remission. Today I saw the nurse practitioner, Marcia, who is petite with short, curly light brown hair and clear, thin glasses. I liked her immediately. She explained that the pet scan showed that I had lesions on my spine, hips, ribs, collarbone and sternum and that she was happy with my bloodwork today. Some of my results had even recovered back to normal range! I had a different nurse take care of me today. She was overly friendly with short dark blonde hair and a pro at administering shots, thus becoming my favorite! I barely felt the prick or the aftermath at all. Later in the day, I wasn't feeling well and had a pounding headache I couldn't seem to make go away. After a three hour nap, I awoke to find Shawn had returned from his work trip. I was overjoyed to see him home. His coworkers had sent him back with a gift basket for me with the most amazingly soft socks, a necklace engraved "LouStrong" and gift cards along with a few other items that I would enjoy.

I had put it off all day, but when it was time for bed, I knew the moment had come. Due to its toxicity, the Revlimid should not be handled, therefore, Shawn emptied a pill into a small clear cup and placed it in my hand. I stared straight through my mother's eyes refusing to break eye contact with her until I started bawling. I was torn between knowing I had to have this medicine to survive and full of fear of all the side effects and secondary cancers this pill brought with it. I eventually slid the blue and white capsule down my throat as the waterworks continued down my pale face. Jean stood strong never breaking eye contact with me, forcing back her own tears until she closed her car door that night to head back home. It broke her to watch me in such peril, wanting so badly to tell me I didn't have to take it and all of this wasn't real. But the reality was, all she could do was stay strong for me in that moment. Shawn slid beside me in bed, where he pulled me close to him smelling my hair laced with coconut shampoo. We had missed each other these last two days. "You have to do this to get better honey and you have to get better because I need you. You are the love of my life and I can't live without you". We both shed a few tears while I lay there on his chest until the ache in my back made me pull away.

It wasn't long before the Revlimid began to wreak havoc on my body. If I didn't think I could feel any worse, I now felt completely terrible. I was so overly tired that I was sleeping the majority of the day. The nausea, the joint aches and there were more bathroom breaks that I cared to endure. Over the last week, I had been doing better walking a little more on my own. I had now backtracked to using my walker full time as my body was reminiscent of a zombie. My medications had caused me to develop

Myopathy, depleting the muscles in my legs, making them sore and weak. I had developed severe acid reflux which had lessened my desire to eat even more. My face, legs, stomach and chest became covered in tiny bright red dots.

Dr. Cawley, in the nicest way possible, explained to me that, unfortunately, I would be feeling this way for a while. She prescribed additional medications in an attempt to reduce the severity of some of my reactions. If the chemo rash did not lessen, it was possible that I may have to reduce my Revlimid dosage. I would have two additional belly shots this cycle to complete the quadrant of red and purple bruises that now covered my bloated stomach.

This cycle had been brutal, however, I can check one more off my countdown. Three more to go.

12

New Normal

One evening I was feeling especially overwhelmed and took to posting on my blog about the magnitude of my daily life. I look back on this post where my words still ring true today.

When I was first diagnosed, the doctors on my team both at home as well as Columbus, kept referring to me living my life as a "new normal". I didn't know what that really meant until this week.

It's taking a plethora of pills three times a day and drinking excessive amounts of water. It's not having an appetite but being urged to eat all the time. It's knowing I have the strength to get through the chemo but being terrified of the upcoming transplant.

It's having to take my temp hourly every chemo shot because my fever spikes in an attempt to avoid a trip back to the hospital because my veins are tired and bruised. It's having one set of pills that make me jittery and awake for twenty-four hours straight and another pill that makes me sleep all day long, giving me terrible nausea and messes with my nerves in my hands and feet. The chemo causes so many issues that the list is never ending. It's having all those side effects, often every day, and your body doesn't know how to react.

It's being thirty-seven years old but using a shower chair and walker (although I'm out of the wheelchair!).

It's being frustrated that you can't do the majority of simple things on your own anymore.

It's thinking I would have all this time to rest, read, watch movies, color, scrapbook, etc., but finding out that instead, my days are filled with appointments, tests, blood work, insurance calls, chemo counseling and so much more. It's being so tired that no amount of sleep seems to awaken me.

It's having chemo brain fog and losing my train of thought mid-sentence. The lack of focus and inability to concentrate tires my mind and overworks my brain causing severe mental fatigue. Multi-tasking becomes non-existent. If I am talking on the phone while cooking, I will most definitely forget an ingredient. Sometimes, I can almost see the words in my head but my brain doesn't connect with my mouth for them to flow out. It's worrying that no matter what I say it won't come out right. I am often scared that my chemo brain will result in dementia, something that broke my heart watching my Mammy battle.

It's trying to figure out how my income has changed and how to pay my son's college tuition, the massive amounts of medical bills coming in and everything else in between.

It's looking in the mirror, seeing how much I have changed and how my belly has went from flat to swollen from the shots.

It's cancelling all the concerts and vacations we had planned this year because they are too risky for me to go. It's not going out into public without wearing a mask. It's getting weird looks because of the cloth covering my face.

It's the Warden sanitizing anyone who comes near me because he needs to protect me.

It's watching my husband hold in his hurt to be my strength. It's knowing my mom has put a hold on her life because she can't stand to not be with me all that she can. It's knowing my son's first year of college is being spent with me on the weekends instead of enjoying his time at school because he thinks he needs to take care of me.

But this is my "new normal" and if this is how it has to be for a year or so then I am lucky that is all it should take to get back to at least a version of my "old normal".

A friend of mine sent me a message the other day: "Psalms 34:18 - The Lord is close to the brokenhearted and saves the crushed in spirit". Through all of this, I have been overwhelmed by so many things. I've have been blessed to have a great marriage that has become so much stronger. All of my friends and family, those close and ones I haven't spoken to in years, have lent support by a prayer, simple message, card, visit, by bringing dinner or sending gifts of love. It's amazing how something so simple can make such a difference to someone in times like these.

So, to all of my family and friends, thank you for lifting my spirits. Thank you for fighting this battle with me. If you work with my husband, thank you for having patience with him. If you are close to my mom, thank you for being there for her as she is having a hard time dealing with this as well.

There is now a commercial for a new medication that plays on television fairly often that includes the phrase "your new normal". Every time I hear it, I still cringe and have now grown to unintentionally mocking it under my breath. *"your new normal"*. I yearn for my "old normal".

13
The James

We had been looking forward to my appointment with the Multiple Myeloma Specialist at the James Cancer Center at Ohio State University in Columbus, Ohio. After the two-hour drive, we arrived at the red brick building towering with glass windows. Immediately upon arrival, I was escorted to the lab to draw blood then wrapped in a lime green bandage. I was accustomed to the drab tan wrap but the nurse explained to me it was fun to have bright colors and it matched the sweatshirt I was wearing, grey with a green outline of our state filled in with flowers. My doctor was a tall, thin man with a dark mustache and wired glasses of Indian descent. He advised us that his name was long and hard to pronounce, therefore, everyone referred to him simply as Dr. D. A FISH panel was a genetic test taken from my biopsy that took weeks to complete. After much anticipation, we were finally getting the results of that test. It was determined that I was of standard risk, stage two out of three. I informed him of the numbness in my hands with concern it was neuropathy, a common side effect from the Velcade. He discussed my upcoming Stem Cell Transplant and all that it would entail at length. I would most likely be admitted to the hospital for two weeks, it would be a miserable ordeal but I would get through it. In order to get the best outcome from it, my Kappa Light Chains would need to decrease by ninety to one hundred percent, however, if my body was unable to reach that goal, it could proceed at fifty percent though the outcome may not be as ideal.

We were told that it is believed that Multiple Myeloma is often found in older men who were exposed to a chemical known as agent orange during Vietnam but that it was possible it could also be from farming chemicals emerged in well water. The mother in me was terrified of it being hereditary, therefore, the possibility of passing it to my child. He assured me that, while some family members share the cancer, it is more likely they had the same exposure, rather than being genetic. Down the road, I would learn that hundreds of people had been diagnosed with Multiple Myeloma from exposure to chemically saturated water on the military base of Camp Lejeune, North Carolina and were being offered compensation for their medical expenses. I had lived there two decades ago, however, the dates that were part of the lawsuit predated my residence there. I suppose we could try to determine how or why I acquired this disease, but in the end, we will never know nor would it change anything. The exciting news was that I was to be studied at Ohio State as part of their research program, therefore, if and when a cure becomes available, I will be one of the first patients contacted.

Shawn and I left The James feeling well educated as well as a little more hopeful. Though unsaid, we were also more fearful of all the transplant would entail. We celebrated the day out by ordering fried macaroni and cheese balls swimming in a mixture of alfredo and marinara along with a decadent dark chocolate cake surrounded in its many layers with light chocolate mousse topped with fresh whipped cream. We enjoyed our date in the parking lot of the Cheesecake Factory using the armrest as our makeshift table. I was exhausted from the magnitude of information and travel the day had held and fell asleep shortly after we pulled on to the interstate.

While most of my bloodwork is resulted within minutes, my light chains and immunoglobulins take longer to return. Later that evening, I answered a phone call from Dr. D, who apologized for the time of the call, though he had been too excited to wait until the next day. In December my Kappas were 4024.0 and today they were 15.0. That was a ninety-six percent decrease. My chemo regimen, terrible as it was, had been successful. The five cycles were now knocked down to only four. I was two down and two more to go in the hopes I would get them down to one hundred percent.

14
The Third Cycle

It was becoming increasingly more difficult to echo "I'm Fine" and maintain my usual essence of positivity. My family had learned to decipher how I was feeling by how my eyes looked that day. Chemo eyes consisted of droopy eyelids, the brightness disappearing with a sickly halo of darkness overtaking my once shiny green eyes. I had tried to stay positive the best I could to make it easier on my loved ones. They lived in a new state of constant worry about my health. Over the last week I have only been eating my mom's homemade noodles and McDonald's hot fudge sundaes. My hands have become so shaky that getting food from the bowl into my mouth is quite the challenge. I might as well forget soup all together. Nonetheless, I forge ahead, though only half the spoonful makes it to its destination. My mother watches in horror, unsure of whether or not she should offer to help me, or if in doing so she will insult my determination. In one instance, watching my noodles slide off on to the counter, she broke her strength, sobbing silently. When it was only the two of us, Shawn would offer to feed me. Sometimes, I would reluctantly give in, too tired to try, but other times, tears would flow, mortified of the situation. On top of that, the chemo caused my skin to crack and itch, becoming painful and irritating. I had begun a rotation of my soft and colorful Cuddl Dud pajamas, only changing into real clothes when I left the house.

Several of my family and friends went together to deliver me a vase full of branches with gift cards for groceries and gas tied on with burgundy ribbon, named the "LouStrong Tree". It was a generous, heartwarming surprise, which was greatly appreciated. All of the ladies at a hair salon in town stayed late one night to put on a "Hair-A-Thon" to see how many haircuts they could complete in one evening. They gave their time for donations only, all of which they presented to Caleb the next day. It was such an honor to have so many people rally around me in our small town including several I had never even had the privilege of meeting.

During my off week, I was blessed with a couple of days where I felt a little better. Over his objections, I was able to do some of Caleb's laundry, as well as make a couple meals for him to take back to school. I know he is capable of doing these tasks himself, but it was important to me to be able to still do some 'mom duties' whenever I was able.

Dr. Cawley met me with exciting news the first day back this cycle beaming with the news that Dr. D. shared with her his belief that I am ahead of schedule, leaving only two more cycles to go! One of the best qualities about her is that she genuinely celebrates the good news with you as well as feels the hurt of the bad news. Today I have a new nurse, the only one wearing a long skirt and brown hair tied up in a bun on top of her head. I enjoy her kindness as well as her gentle hand stinging my belly. In order to lessen the pain, my shots are rotated in quadrants around my stomach in the hopes my bruises will begin healing in those areas by the next cycle. The good nurses, who warm the syringe first with their hands and inject it slowly, leave smaller pink roses, whereas, the other nurses are quick to shove it in and move on. Those areas inflate to deep purple painful expansions that take over my abdomen.

I arrived to my appointment on Valentine's Day, wearing a lavender hoodie, white floral leggings and skipping my usual double braids to leave my hair down, covered with a light grey hat with tiny white flowers. I was immediately presented with gifts made for the cancer patients from local elementary school students. They included a blue heart ornament with foam stickers that spelled out LOVE, lip balm, a box of candy hearts, a crayon drawing of a rainbow as well as a pink construction paper card covered in artwork of hearts and colored arches with well wishes to have a great day. I was smitten with these children who took great pride in the gifts they had made to brighten someone's day without knowing them. Today I was anxious about receiving my first infusion of a bone strengthener called Zometa. Though it was given to help repair the holes chiseled out of my bones, I had read that it also came with debilitating bone pain for a few days thereafter. As I lay reclined in my tan leather chair, as a new drug traveling through my veins was slowly being released from the clear bag hanging from the pole, I gazed at my husband sitting across from me who gave me a wink. My eyes moved past him to the sun shining against the window from the clear blue sky which had been dreary and grey the last few days. Despite everything, I was blessed.

I woke up in the middle of the night ravaging in pain. Every bone in my body was screaming from my skull to my toes. Shawn wrapped me in a cocoon in my sherpa heated blanket whispering that I was going to be okay. This was a new ache. A new, excruciating ache radiating through every bone in my body. Another medicine given to help me heal that seemed to bring along additional side effects to add to my ever-growing list. After realizing my Oxycodone would not be a remedy for my current agony, a quick call to the nurse line suggested I try taking Claritin. Sounds weird right? For whatever reason, this antihistamine provided a bit of relief for my bone pain over the next couple of days, just enough to cut the edge. I was supposed to schedule this torture every other month for two years. Going forward, I would be given a similar drug known as Xgeva, due to my inability to tolerate the Zometa. Although still extremely uncomfortable, it was better than its predecessor.

By the time my third cycle was over, I was grateful my five cycles had been changed to four and I was ready to push forward.

15

The Benefit

Last month, my friend Beth, together with Megan and her sister-in-law, Heather, shared with me they were preparing to organize a benefit to help lessen the burden of my overwhelming pile of medical bills. Within ten weeks, I had already racked up seventy-three claims. At first, Shawn and I were uncomfortable with the idea of accepting money from friends and family, but eventually agreed on the offer. The soup and salad dinner was set apart from the usual spaghetti benefits in our town and would be held at a local school cafeteria. Although I was the guest of honor, my doctors rejected the idea of me attending due to my weakened immune system. When the day arrived, I snuck into the venue for just a few minutes, taken aback by what I saw. Burgundy flowers and coordinating tablecloths decorated with bundles of balloons spread across the vast gymnasium floor. One entire wall was filled with tables overflowing with silent auction items. A backdrop stood near the door next to a bin full of cancer related photo props encouraging guests to partake. Pictures of me from both before and after my diagnosis lined the walls, hanging from tiny clothespins on a clear thread. The aroma of freshly prepared soup warming in dozens of crock pots filled the air and consisted of vegetable, potato and chili, among others. In honor of my recent cravings, a variety of marshmallow crispy treats covered the dessert area. I was overwhelmed by the generosity from those who had donated their time, food and supplies to support me.

Those who had already arrived were all wearing LouStrong shirts. As hungry guests began signing the register at the doorway, Shawn had to pull me away. Every part of my being wanted to stay and socialize. I craved human interaction. I have always been the person who loves family get togethers, mostly in part due to growing up close to my wonderful aunts and uncles. To me, this occasion felt the same way.

A few weeks ago, a photographer friend of mine offered to gift a photo shoot before I went for transplant and lost my hair. She had already shot some of Shawn, Joey and I on the farm. It was raw, emotional and surrounded by fields of hay, still scarce from the winter. I also wanted family pictures, but needed to wait until Shawn's parents, as well as my brother and his wife, were here. Everyone had arrived for the big event today, so we spread out, my closest family and my best friend, across a railroad track right down from the school, dressed in grey and burgundy butterfly shirts, holding hands side by side.

I drove home, heart warmed from all the love I felt tonight in just the few short minutes I had been a part of it, but also with my heart aching that I wasn't able to stay. Shawn carried "Facetime Me" on the iPad around that evening to allow me to feel as if I were there. This made an initially sad evening fun and exciting. It was obvious that everyone there was having an amazing time. Guests were smiling and laughing, enjoying socialization with one another. I spoke to many of my loved ones, making sure to express my gratitude to each new face on my screen. My husband, who felt awkward about the situation at the beginning, was now overwhelmed by the amount of love pouring out that night. His immense gratitude could be felt by the tears welling up in his blue eyes as he gave a thank you speech that evening.

A couple of days later, Beth, my sassy, good hearted, decades long friend, stopped by with the donations, along with a gift basket overflowing with items I may need in the upcoming months. After passing the Warden's preliminary test, we chatted at length about old times while watching me try on caps as we pulled the different colored cotton wraps from the bin one after another. The escapade filled us both with much needed laughter.

.

16

The Fourth Cycle

The dates for my Preliminary Testing, Stem Cell Harvest, as well as my Transplant have been set. Three major milestones to complete. I have an ever-growing list that needs accomplished but I am aware these next few weeks will move by quickly. Although Shawn would prefer that we don't discuss the possibility of my mortality, I have been diligent in ensuring that all of my estate affairs have been updated. There is a binder containing spreadsheets of our bills and passwords along with pages of all the health and insurance information. I felt better knowing that, if I am incapacitated, these things will be easily accessible.

During the first appointment of my fourth cycle, Dr. Cawley shares with me that, as long as my doctor at the James is agreeable, this shall be the final two weeks of my initial treatment! While I had anticipated this news after my last visit to Ohio State, there was still the possibility my numbers wouldn't support it. Today is also the fitting for my free wig that is donated to each cancer patient ahead of impending baldness. This was one thing I hadn't come to terms with yet. I was terrified of saying goodbye to my long blonde curls. Standing outside the room lined with plastic mannequins topped with a variety of hair styles and colors, I took a deep breath before stepping through the doorway. To my disappointment, we were unable to find one that resembled my hair, but I settled on a darker blonde, shoulder length wig with thick curls. It would do for now.

My Myeloma Specialist was impressed with how quickly I responded to treatment as well as how I completed in only four cycles. We discussed at length what the two days of testing I would have to endure next week would entail. These evaluations would determine if I was strong enough for transplant. It sounds brutal and exhausting but I was ready to power through it all.

March 14, 2019 would be my last day of treatment for my initial regimen. The final prick of Velcade inserted into my sore belly. To celebrate this victory, I would wear my LouStrong shirt, burgundy bracelet and double braided hair. Even after this, I will still receive my bone strengthener every other month for nearly two years. But today, I will be escorted by my favorite nurse to the large brass bell attached to the wall where she will throw her arms around me in excitement. "Congratulations! It's your last day! It's your turn to ring the bell" she exclaims. For a moment, the world stood still as I took the fraying rope in my hand then shook it back and forth. The room erupted with applause. I could feel the tears burning in the corners of my eyes as I smiled sheepishly, embarrassed being the center of attention. Relief that I was finishing a milestone. Fear of what was to come. Empathy for those celebrating me sitting in cubicles with bags of chemicals flowing through their veins. Some would have better outcomes than me, others worse. Grateful beyond measure for the medical care I had been given here. Then, I caught a glance of my husband's eyes, where tears glassed over his baby blues. Beaming with pride for the strength it took from me to make it to this day.

Although often difficult to maneuver without pain, I have also graduated from my walker this week! Additionally, this accomplishment gives me the freedom to shower on my own, though still requiring the chair as well as hand rails. Being able to close my eyes and relax while letting the steaming water trickle all around me without my mother or husband keeping a watchful eye, fearful I may fall, was liberating.

As I began to prepare for transplant, I would get a break from my chemo medications, so that my body may have an opportunity to regain strength. I looked forward to the possibility of a couple of weeks of "normality". The calm before the storm.

17

Forty-Eight Hours

An overwhelming sense of fear and determination overcame me as we pulled in to the James just as the sun was peaking over the horizon. I held in my hand a two-page typed evaluation schedule for the next couple of days along with a gallon size jug filled to the brim with the last twenty-four hours of my bodily fluids. The first day, the easier of the two, consisted of an Echocardiogram to determine if my heart was strong enough to proceed.

We were given a white binder filled with page after page of all the information we would need to prepare for the upcoming transplant. Accompanying these instructions would be a slide show as well as a movie covering all the basics. "This will be rough. Really rough. You WILL be miserable for a while and you need to be prepared" my doctor reiterated. Was I? Mentally, I was ready to conquer another milestone. But emotionally, I was petrified. To date, there was never a moment where I was angry over my situation. There had been plenty of occasions where I felt defeated, sad, lonely, but I could not change my diagnosis. Being mad at my situation would do nothing but waste the little energy I maintained. All I could do was move forward with a positive outlook, graduating from one milestone to another.

We continued the afternoon by visiting the social worker and transplant coordinator. One of the exams I was most anxious about was to determine if my veins were strong enough to withstand the enormous steel needles used to harvest my stem cells. I had always been blessed with large veins, however, they had whittled away during my stay in the hospital. The alternative was to have a port placed in the side of my neck, the thought of which frightened me. Thankfully, my veins had recovered to the point in which the doctor felt they would be viable for harvest.

The next morning began with pulmonary testing, followed by a chest x-ray, as well as a Myeloma Survey, also known as Skeletal Survey. It consists of a collection of x-rays inclusive of all bones in entirety to assess any further damage or new lesions. This survey is essential in patients with Non-Secretory Myeloma, such as myself.

Day two also consisted of the more difficult testing. It began with extracting twenty-two vials of blood in order to create a baseline. Transplants held the capability to alter my body in mysterious ways including the occasional blood type change. In nearly all cases, all childhood vaccines are evaporated, thus needing to be re-administered for two years post-transplant. The nurse was impressed with my ability to keep from fainting while she was draining me of what felt like my entire blood supply. I would then move on to an EKG, followed by a physical exam by my doctor.

On to the last procedure, the one I was looking forward to the least, another bone marrow biopsy. Lying on a gurney, steel bars surrounding me as if I had planned to escape, my body felt the pure exhaustion hovering from the last two days. Behind a closed grey curtain hanging in the doorway, my husband kissed my forehead, reminding me that we were nearing the end of this endeavor. It wasn't long before the doctor pushed a cocktail of Morphine and Ativan through my IV. Laying on my side, my eyes widened when the world's largest syringe accompanied by an equally frightening needle began its way in to my bone marrow via my hip. I could feel my eyes cringe, glaring at the man in the white coat. I felt the pain taking over my body but at the same time the drugs made me feel as if I didn't care. What a strange out of body experience. The feeling of agony and indifference at the same time. When the procedure was complete, the portal to my veins was removed from my arm then wrapped in bright red to match my Ohio State shirt.

I am a bit of a lightweight when it comes to medications, thus, I don't remember much of the trip back home. My husband tells me I had made up my mind that I needed to stop for Dibs, the little bite size pieces of creamy vanilla ice cream covered in crispy chocolate coating. When we stopped for gas shortly after departing the hospital, I meandered the aisles in search of my craving. Shawn suggested we may have to look elsewhere, unsure if a convenience store would carry such a product. Forty-five minutes later, due to my incoherent state of wandering, I handed this patient man of mine the small red pint-sized container. "See, I told you they had Dibs" I stated as I wandered off to the car while he paid the cashier. Proud of myself, for I showed him. To this day, he still finds this recollection hilarious.

At the end of these last two days of evaluations, I received two notifications. I had been cleared for transplant and I had achieved complete response. There is no cure for Multiple Myeloma, therefore, the word "remission" is a term that can be hoped for but never spoken. This was the best outcome I could have wished for, however, deep down I knew my battle was still only beginning. I would always be a passenger on a roller coaster of highs and lows.

18

Birthday Harvest

I had hoped that being off the chemo in preparation for transplant would bring a rejuvenation of normality but I had been suffering from the debilitating pain associated with the bone strengthener. I was no longer taking the high dose steroid that assisted in masking some of the anguish. Even the Oxycodone failed to bring relief. I felt defeated and frustrated.

My brother and his wife came down for the weekend to celebrate our birthdays a little early this year. Caleb was my April Fool's Day baby and my birthday followed his by two days. My gift from Shawn and Caleb was a photo shoot in our fancy attire. A perfect gift for me. I wore my sparkly, navy blue lace dress that I had purchased specifically to wear to the Hamilton play and the boys looked dapper in their crisp blue suits.

I have always been known as a fixer. I have an overwhelming need to make life easier for others. On top of that, I felt as if my mothering duties had been lost over these last few months. I was determined to ensure my husband and my son would be taken care of during my recovery, both of whom could easily provide for themselves, but I still felt they were my responsibility. Knowing I would no longer be able to complete the task on my own, I enlisted Megan to assist me in stocking our freezer with enough meals, both regular as well as vegan, to nourish them during my absence. After an entire day of cooking, the freezer was filled to capacity, stocked with casseroles, soups and family favorites, ensuring my boys would have a hot meal every night.

During a Bone Marrow Transplant, stem cells are extracted from the bone marrow. A Stem Cell Transplant is now more widely used due to the fact the stem cells can be used from the more easily accessible bloodstream. When I was first diagnosed, many of my family members, as well as a client from the law office, were the first to volunteer to be tested as a possible donor match for my transplant. Though humbled by their gestures, I was lucky enough to be able to do an Autologous Stem Cell Transplant, which meant I could use my own stem cells. In order to increase and mobilize them out of my bone marrow and into my bloodstream, it was necessary for me to resume belly shots. I would need injections of Neupogen, a colony stimulator, every morning at home for five days. Shawn was increasingly nervous about hurting me, but he actually did a really good job pricking my stomach with the tiny needles. Forcing my body to rapidly increase my white blood cells by kicking my bone marrow into overdrive brought about a level of pain far worse than even my bone strengthener. As I struggled through the agony that I was attempting to hide as a show of strength for my already overly worried family, I watched the clock eagerly, desperately waiting for each time I could have another dose of Claritin and narcotics. I was naïve in thinking that my anguished face could mask this amount of nagging pain but, per usual, I insisted I was fine.

The stars had aligned the day before my harvest. Much to everyone's frustration, Shawn had to attend a mandatory two-day work conference in Columbus. It just so happened that Al also had to be up there the following two days for an Ohio Farm Bureau meeting. Therefore, it worked out well to ride up with Al and meet Shawn in Columbus. That morning, it was Al's duty to inject me with more mobilizers. Being accustomed to frequently giving the cattle shots, he stuck my belly with ease. My mom spent the morning showering me with birthday gifts that included a mug stating that I, in fact, was the favorite child, an ongoing banter between my brother and me. Then, after an embrace I was sure she was not going to release, Al and I departed, watching tears roll down her face in the rearview mirror. A mother's worry for all that her daughter was about to endure was obvious.

Shortly after arriving through the vast atrium of the ground floor of the James, my brother arrived to relieve Al of his caretaker duties, however, he decided to opt out of his luncheon to stay with me during my testing. He snapped a photo of me in a floral shirt under a lilac cardigan, hands in my denim pockets, leaning against the wall underneath the heading "Hematology & Transplant". Al has a passion for taking photos just as much as I do. During my evaluation a couple of weeks ago, my white blood count was 4.94. It was now 60.83. The exorbitant amount of pain I had endured this week from the mobilizers had been worth it. I was cleared for harvest. As we were finishing up my appointment, Shawn had made it just in time. We said goodbye to Al as he left for his work obligations, then my brother escorted me to the car, his hand in mine, where we all headed to the Hobby Lobby. At the time, we did not have my favorite store in our hometown, so visiting it was an absolute necessity. I can't say that the guys loved spending their afternoon at a craft store, but they found enjoyment hiding in between hanging greenery and being silly to lighten the mood we were all feeling inside. After our shopping trip, we went back to Chad's house to clean up before dinner. I walked in to find purple and teal balloons topped with a sign that read "Happy Birthday", decorated by my sister-in-law. I was turning thirty-eight years old today. We celebrated with dinner at O'Charleys, where it was free pie Wednesday. Being that the boys don't share my love of sweets, they gifted me their slices. I settled on cherry, creamy butterscotch topped with a healthy dollop of whipped cream, and frozen strawberry with cookie crust. Being completely drained afterward, Shawn and I headed back to the hotel for a good night's rest. His managers, who I also consider part of our family, had sent me a care package with him after their conference that included cards full of love and well wishes along with gifts of faith and encouragement. Though not how I had planned to spend my birthday, this was a great surprise to finish out the evening.

I awoke the next morning ready to conquer yet another milestone of this journey I had now found myself on. Dressed in my signature LouStrong shirt and double braids, we set out on our next adventure. When we arrived, a young nurse, new to this position, explained to us how the massive machine sitting in the middle of my room would perform a procedure called Apheresis, meaning "to take away". A regular IV would be placed in one arm along with a larger IV catheter inserted with a wider steel needle in the other. Nurses have typically been fond of the vein in my right arm due to its size, making it easily accessible. My first thought was that the larger needle would be inserted in that more predominant vein. The nurse disagreed, noting that one was further away from the machine. She failed miserably, and painfully, at getting the giant steel needle into my smaller vein. My arm was already beginning to turn into a blotch of dark purple bruises. The Warden was becoming increasingly irritated at her incompetence. At some point, she left the room, only to return with an older nurse, who was infuriated with the current state of my veins. Within minutes, a myriad of tubes were flowing out of both arms into the contraption beside my bed. The new nurse rotated heat packs on my busted arm that now appeared to have several tentacles flowing from my veins.

Due to my current attachment, bathroom privileges were forbidden, so I passed on eating lunch even though it would have filled the time. We were quickly engaged in watching the Apheresis machine do its work. My blood would flow out of one tube straight into the machine which would then separate out the stem cells from my blood, returning only a small amount of blood back into my body. It was fascinating to watch modern medical science perform in all its glory.

Five and a half hours later, I was discharged from the hospital with the promise we wouldn't leave town until we were called with my results. If I had been unsuccessful in harvesting enough stem cells, I would have to repeat the process again tomorrow. By the looks of the growing contusions around my veins, I was unsure how that would even be possible. My body was exhausted. All I wanted to do was go home and crawl in my own pillow soft bed. I needed to quench my thirst since I had been dry for the last several hours for fear of the bed pan. We stopped at a nearby restaurant for a drink, and to this day, I still remember the satisfaction of that ice cold tea kissed with a hint of peach. My body was so worn down that I was unsure if I had the capability of walking, let alone shopping, but I've never passed up an opportunity to check out a new T.J. Maxx and there was one right there staring at me. We had just walked through the automatic doors, arm in arm, as I wasn't stable enough to move forward on my own, when my phone rang. The goal was to collect five million stem cells, which would be divided equally. Half to be utilized for this transplant, the remainder to be frozen and stored for another one. I had harvested 9.26 million stem cells! I was homebound.

Jean had gifted me a foot spa for my birthday. She was at my house waiting for me when we returned home, the small tub filled with water bubbling away. After a little assistance making my way over to the sofa, I let out a long sigh of relief as my tired calves slid in to the warm water.

The last feat before transplant: complete.

19

Preparing for Transplant

A common side effect of the Velcade is Chemo Induced Peripheral Neuropathy which damages healthy nerves. Immediately after harvest, what had started as numbness in my hands a few weeks ago, had escalated to my feet. What felt like constant bee stings, my toe nails slowly being ripped from my skin and shooting sharp pains from my toes up my legs, was unbearable. Seriously? Haven't I endured enough pain? Neuropathy tends to be worse at night, when I would spend countless hours bawling. At this point, I think of myself fairly pain tolerant, as I have learned to live daily life with constant discomfort, but this was pure torture. Pain meds were useless. Heat provided some relief, thus being the beginning of my continuous life under a heated blanket, which I later deemed a fix for all things. My doctor increased my daily intake of Gabapentin in the hopes it would make the pain tolerable.

I had been advised it would be best if I cut my hair shorter prior to transplant but had been putting it off for quite some time now. I had made up my mind that I would get mermaid hair, an ombre effect of my favorite colors, teal, purple and green, prior to letting it go. In the end, I decided that it was a waste of money to color my hair just to lose it. A decision I would later regret and vow to do if I ever were in this situation again. My hair stylist was my cousin, who offered to complete this unwanted task at my home, hoping to make the process a little easier for me. She cut it off from a braid, which I still keep in a small box of cancer mementos that I hold on to reminisce from time to time. I couldn't watch my blonde curls fall to the floor so she was quick to sweep them up before handing me the mirror. To my surprise, my new look was cute! My hair landed just below my ears, making my wavy curls appear much thicker now. To celebrate, Jean took me to Dairy Queen, where over the last several weeks I had grown quite fond of a mixture of chocolate and vanilla soft serve covered in cherry coating. This treat had served as my dinner on several occasions. She purchased two quarts of the swirled ice cream then sweet talked the manager in to selling her a container of the cherry topping so that I would be stocked at home during my post-transplant quarantine.

Still not willing to give up my fixer status, I had been putting together gift baskets for Shawn, as well as Mom and Al. At first, they were unsure of how to react. I was the one going through this life changing procedure, yet I needed to do what I could for them to make their lives easier for the next few weeks while boring themselves watching me in the hospital. My parents' tote included comfy socks, word puzzles, books, a variety of snacks since Jean gets hangry, as well as other items to keep them occupied during travel and visits. Shawn's basket consisted of iced coffee, beef jerky, a variety of hunting and fishing magazines as well as fun items adorned with sticky notes. His favorite photo of me from our wedding "in case you forget what I looked like with hair". A package of cinnamon hard candies "because I think you're hot". If nothing else, I hoped these gifts would lift their spirits. I needed to make sure these people who have been by my side taking care of me the last few months were taken care of too. I didn't have a lot to give right now other than my unconditional love and appreciation.

The night before we were due to check in at the James was spent preparing for the days ahead. I finished packing my new, freshly washed pajamas that were required to be v-neck for easier access to the port that would be placed inside my chest. Remembering just how uncomfortable hospital bedding can be, I set out my own pillow, along with extra pillowcases, bright white with little turquoise flowers, knowing that it would be necessary to replace them daily. A bag was filled with books and word puzzles to occupy my time as well as the Roku stick for the TV, with the intent of being able to catch up on Game of Thrones.

After showering, Shawn assisted me in wiping myself down with the special disinfecting sheets I had been instructed to use. We spent the rest of the evening cuddled up together in bed, Joey's furry little head resting on my chest. Nerves were taking over, but as I drifted off to sleep that night, I remember my husband kissing me on the forehead, whispering "I got you baby".

20
Transplant

The positivity I had tried so incredibly hard to maintain over the last four months was fading. Fear had taken over. I had been warned that going through transplant would be my hardest battle thus far. I have always admired my husband's hands, strong yet soft, showing years of hard work, and mine would stay intertwined with his the entire two hour car ride and until we stepped foot off the elevator to the fifteenth floor.

One must acquire special access in order to be allowed on the transplant floor. Everyone is required to wear N95 masks and visitations are limited. This ward has a separate ventilation system, blowing in cooler air, which was essential in preventing infections. The linens are changed and rooms are sanitized daily. The faint aroma of bleach filled the air. My new sterile abode was rather large for a hospital room and included a full bathroom, complete with my own shower. A reclining chair sat in the corner next to the bed. A small sofa made of fake plastic leather was positioned underneath a large window overlooking a breathtaking view of the skyscrapers towering over downtown Columbus. My digital frame was set up beside the bed, allowing me to feel more at home as my most cherished photographs rotated throughout the day.

Soon after we arrived, I was whisked away downstairs to an operating room so that a Central Venous Catheter port could be surgically inserted into the large vein just above my heart. Shortly after the nurse had pushed anesthesia through my veins, the surgeon hovered over top of me preparing to make the incision. "Ummm should I still be awake?" I questioned, which resulted in more sedation chemicals to be administered. Three more times. Still awake. Finally, a numbing shot was slipped in to my chest. I returned to my room with an abundance of plastic tubes sewn into my body. As inconvenient as it would be trying to maneuver without tugging on them, which I quickly found out could be quite uncomfortable, the port would make life much easier to extract blood, as well as administer all the medications I would surely need. Once back in my room, I was allowed to change out of the hospital gown that had been several sizes too big for me and into my new navy blue Cuddl Duds. The shorts and button up top were covered in bright pink and aqua flowers all trimmed in white. If I was going to be stuck in a sterile room for the next several days, I may as well look cute.

Melphalan is a strong, nasty form of chemotherapy. It is so powerful I would only need one infusion prior to transplant. It is used to wipe clean any residual myeloma cells in preparation for the re-infusion of the harvested stem cells, which in turn rescue the bone marrow from the effects of this chemo. Of all the medications I had endured over the last several months, this one treatment would be all it would take to destroy my hair. This drug was also known to cause raw, painful sores in the mouth. In an attempt to combat this awful side effect, it was necessary for me to eat ice for two full hours before it was to be administered. Cup after cup overflowing with cold crushed ice was ushered to me throughout the evening. It didn't take long for me to dislike the spoonfuls of frozen water being shoveled into my mouth and held there until almost melted, then finally allowed to move down my throat. Although I was covered in a mountain of blankets, I was freezing. I couldn't stop shivering. Knowing the alternative, I was determined to power through the next two hours, encouraging Shawn to keep feeding me ice as much as humanly possible. The thought of open sores covering the insides of my mouth was horrifying.

At eleven o'clock that evening my ice consumption was complete. The time had come to administer the Melphalan. My eyes met my husband's when I burst into tears. Everything had come to fruition and emotions came pouring out. I did not want to go through with this transplant. I was tired of having cancer. I needed my hair. I was scared of all that I had been warned I was about to endure. Shawn rested his warm hands around my face reassuring me I was the strongest person he had ever known. We would overcome this hurdle together. He wiped my tears as I gently nodded to the nurse signaling it was okay to plunge the poison into my chest. There would be no turning back now.

Shortly after the clock struck midnight, my eyes rolled back in my head until I lost consciousness. In a panic, Shawn screamed at an orderly nurse passing by in the hallway, who froze, unsure of what he should do to assist me. He ran out of the room to find help. My husband was frantic, shaking me, calling my name. Begging me to wake up. A moment forever embedded in his memory. A nurse practitioner ran in to my room, pushing meds into my tubes, waving alcohol under my nose. I would regain consciousness for a brief moment only to lose it again.

Once I was finally able to stay coherent, the vomiting began, which resulted in more drugs being administered to combat the nausea. Finally stabilized, she explained that the anesthetic (fentanyl) I was given for my port placement was caught up in my IV, then suddenly released all at once. This would also explain why it had not knocked me out earlier during the procedure.

Learning from his stay at Riverside, Shawn came prepared for this getaway by bringing along an inflatable camping mat to lay over his makeshift sofa bed. I referred to it as a raft. That first evening, he laid upon the green waffled topper but he did not sleep. Fearful of what he had witnessed that evening, he took his watch as my protector.

I was told that the first two days I would feel fairly normal and that I should bring things to do to pass the time. Nobody accounted for my drug overdose from the night before. I felt terrible. Although I was being pushed drugs, as well as ingesting a small yellow pill to combat the queasiness, the nausea had overtaken me. Needless to say, my plan to get lost in one of the books I had brought along with me, was foiled. I was also still dealing with the neuropathy in my feet not being controlled. Heating pads were not allowed in hospitals as they posed a fire hazard. The nurses were constantly laying small white heating packs on my angry toes which would provide relief for only a few minutes until they cooled down. Eventually, I was offered a blanket attached by a hose to a water heater. Once it bubbled and heated up it was supposed to provide warmth to the blanket. It left a lot to be desired.

April 17, 2019. Transplant Day. A day that is referred to as my "Re-Birthday". It is a day to celebrate. The nutrition staff brought in cheesecake decorated with raspberry compote that read "Happy Transplant Day". It was accompanied by a card with a thumbs up smiling emoji signed by all my medical staff. Though I was still unable to keep anything down in my stomach, the gesture, along with the enthusiasm for the day, was well appreciated. I was wearing my soft and cozy Lion King shirt, which read "Hakuna Matata". Jean and Al were there to celebrate the occasion with me. The Stem Cell Transplant itself was fairly uneventful. We were all required to be dressed in hospital gowns, latex gloves, a hair covering that resembled a shower cap and the world's most suffocating masks attached by two thick rubber bands. A large white cooler was wheeled in on top of a stainless cart. The clear bag containing my stem cells is hung on the pole beside my bed and connected to my port for distribution. An hour later, my transplant was complete. We had been warned, but I don't think anyone could anticipate, just how strange it would be to smell like creamed corn, an odor specific to the solution my stem cells had been bathing in the last couple of weeks.

Later that day, my brother came to visit and accompanied me on my twice daily mandatory walks down the hallway, while dragging my pole adorned with a myriad of clear bags and being forced to wear the airless duck mask. He walked tall beside me, my arm intertwined in his, my weak body slowly growing closer to him as we meandered down the quiet sterile corridor.

Since I had apparently found myself celebrating holidays in the hospital this year, Easter was no exception.

I was offered a special dinner, one that I would have to decline. Other than the occasional chocolate Frosty, I had been too nauseas to eat. Five days after transplant, my white blood cells bottomed out to zero. My immune system was officially decimated. My body felt as if I had a boulder pushing down on me. I was so weak that the mere thought of getting out of bed was exhausting. Ignoring my objections, my medical staff required that I roam the halls twice a day. The duck mask made it impossible to breathe through the exertion it would take for me to force my legs to move. Shawn held me up on one side as I pulled along my lifeline pole on the other. My shower routine was even worse. Keeping in line with the other daily sterilizing routines, it was mandated that I shower once a day. A nurse would help me undress, cover me in plastic wrap to protect my port and wash me as I rested on a bench while warm water glided over me. Annoyed by this entire process, after a few days, I finally convinced the nurse to allow my husband to bathe me instead. Following my shower, along with two other times each day, I was required to use a special mouthwash. There were two plastic tubes that were mixed together upon opening. Being nauseas already, the minty concoction was less than desirable. Every transplant patient has to deal with loose stools. Even more exciting, is that the nurses have to look at them every time I went to the bathroom to make sure I did not have C. Diff or other infection. I was quickly made aware that I would have no privacy during my stay. Countless nurses had seen me naked and examined my bowel movements. At this point, I was so miserable that I didn't even care.

I had been successful in my ice usage and thankfully did not have to deal with mouth sores. I did, however, manage to get a sort of freezer burn instead. To combat this, I was given large white tablets to dissolve in my mouth three times a day which made my nausea worse. On several occasions, I would hide them in the cart beside my bed. Shawn would eventually find them a couple days later. Sorry, not sorry. I hated them. Between the Ativan and the Compazine, my nausea drug, all I wanted to do is sleep. Every four hours, a nurse would appear to take my vitals and draw blood, along with the occasional doctor visit in between. I was constantly being stuck in the stomach with shots to prevent blood clots, so much so, that there were a few days that Shawn refused to let them prick me, just to give me a break.

At one point, my platelets dropped to a mere six and I began receiving platelet and blood infusions, which would continue over the next few days. One day, I spiked a fever, along with a drop in my blood pressure, causing my medical staff to begin a frenzy of testing. Having absolutely no immune system, one doctor reminded us that they needed to move quickly because any infection could kill me. Something as simple as a single mold spore could take over my entire body.

This would also be the same day my hair started falling out in wide chunks. The texture had grown rough and brittle in just a few days. It was destroyed by the poison ravaging through my body. Apparently, this was all I needed to see in order to be ready to let it all go. Shortly thereafter, I asked a nurse to shave my head. Looking at myself in the mirror afterward, I felt a sense of relief. No crying. No more fear of not having it. There would be no mistaking me for anyone other than a cancer patient. I was bald. To be honest, in my current state, it was more comfortable than having to deal with hair in my face. My husband truly saw me no differently. He loved me with all his heart, hair or no hair.

After fifteen days of surviving in the sterile transplant ward, my numbers began increasing and I was discharged. When the doctor came in to remove my port, I was given two options: a Lidocaine shot around the area or just "rip it out". I had enough shots this week so I timidly went for option two. Hovering over top me, she instructed me to hold my breath as she extracted the tentacles from my body. It was the strangest sensation I had ever felt. As if my chest opened up and ejected the never-ending wires that had been my lifeline the last several days, replenishing my body with whatever was needed. Within seconds they were gone.

Before I was able to depart, we were given several pages of instructions of what not to do over the next one hundred days. All my toiletries were required to be hypoallergenic. It was forbidden to be around real flowers or any type of gardening, as they could contain harmful bacteria spores. Foods such as deli meats, eggs that were not fully cooked, sushi and raw honey were not allowed. My bedding needed to be changed daily. My childhood vaccines had been depleted; therefore, I had no protection from illnesses such as measles and chicken pox. I was also severely immunocompromised on top of everything else. A mask was required anywhere I went but it was suggested I stay home over the next several months.

When she was not visiting me at the James, my mother had been working diligently to sanitize our home. I am certain that my house had never been this clean. Every room was bleached and sanitized from top to bottom. All the curtains and linens had been washed. The filters changed. An ozone generator ran for days to kill any remaining germs. Jean had worked tirelessly for two weeks to ensure I would return to a clean home, free of anything in the air that may harm me. Simply put, my mom is the best.

Shawn rolled up the raft that he had called his bed over the last couple of weeks. Although I missed out due to my constant state of sleep, he was able to catch up on multiple seasons of Game of Thrones. He had brought his laptop, enabling him to continue working, but I am positive he was overcome with boredom. Jean and Al had offered to stay overnight with me so he could get a good night's sleep at a nearby hotel that I could see from the window. Just like my stay in Riverside, my husband refused to leave my side, even though it required him to wear a mask the entire stay. He never once complained. I don't know what I did to deserve this amazing, loyal, patient man of mine, but I am forever grateful to have been blessed with him in my life.

The time had come. Too weak to walk long distances, I was brought down to our mocha-colored GMC Acadia in a wheelchair, a black cap with mint green flowers protecting my newly bald head. In two short hours, I would be back home.

21

One Hundred Days

The aroma of the fresh scent of Lysol surrounded us the moment we came through the door. Jean had outdone herself. I was sure my house would never be this sterile again. After a hot shower, once again being monitored and requiring assistance, I slid into my freshly washed, crisp sheets, nuzzling my face down into my cozy tower of pillows. I had missed the warmth and relief of the heated sherpa blanket. I was sound asleep within seconds. There is nothing better than sleeping in your own bed. It was required that I have a caregiver with me around the clock. My mom had resumed staying here until bedtime, which left Al and Megan to babysit me while Shawn and Jean were at work. Every time I would need to go to the restroom or take a shower, I would return to the bedroom, only to find the bed had been made, blankets turned down on my side, inviting me back in. That was my mother, always taking care of me.

My body was increasingly weak. My appetite was non-existent. Between all the weight I had shed in the hospital and the massive amount of muscle loss, Shawn joked that my calves appeared to have water balloons hanging from them. Joking aside, losing muscle is incredibly painful. Walking to another room or even picking up a dinner plate took effort. I shriveled away to a little over one hundred pounds, down nearly twenty less than my normal weight, with sunken eyes surrounded by darkness and a bald head. The reflection staring back at me in the mirror was not me. I saw a weak, frail alien full of anguish.

Though I had been instructed not to let Joey return home for thirty days, I could no longer bear him not being here with me. Five days after returning home, ignoring my parents' insistence that he remain with them, my furry faced bundle of joy came beaming through the front door straight to the bedroom. Shawn scooped him up before he could jump on the bed, annoying him with a thorough wipe down first. His puppy eyes with a human softness seemed to understand as I explained to him, though I wanted nothing more, he wasn't allowed to shower me with kisses for the time being. My protector twirled in a circle, then found his place in the back of my knees, where he would remain until I moved. My heart was content now that we were all under one roof.

One week later at my follow up appointment, my doctor expressed his displeasure about my continuing weight loss, insisting that I try protein shakes, at the very least. I enjoy most foods, but I despise milk products, with the exception of ice cream, meaning shakes were out of the question. I was already dealing with enough nausea. My blood pressure was low, causing me to receive an infusion of fluids. At home, I can whine to my mom that I don't feel like eating and she just says "ok honey, you don't have to eat", whereas the boys force me to take a few bites. I started referring to Caleb as "Warden Jr." They all took fantastic care of me in their own way. My son showed me a video of a final project he submitted at college. It begins with "And she loved a little boy very, very much, even more than she loved herself", a quote from his favorite book as a child, The Giving Tree, by

Shel Silverstein. His sweet smile spreads nervously across his face as he goes on to share examples of how selfless of a mother that he believed I was, noting that I was the strongest person he knew. I am touched by the sentiment and so incredibly proud of my child.

Since transplant, I have struggled with not being able to sleep. I'm lucky if I get four hours throughout the night. Exhaustion has taken over me. My body needs sleep to recover. I become beyond frustrated and beg my doctors to fix my insomnia. The pain in my muscles and joints has worsened when I had hoped it would ease over time. Most annoying, is that my neuropathy is still not under control.

In an attempt to lighten everyone's mood, including my own, I took to Snapchat to create a video, while singing "Nothing Compares to You" by Sinead O'Connor, changing the words as I saw fit for my current situation. I was sporting a gold nose ring and dark lipstick which gave my family a good laugh. The following day, my brother was graduating from college, officially titled as Nurse Practitioner. Unable to attend, I sent in my place an enlarged photo of myself, crystal tiara on top of my head, taped to a wooden paint stick. As Chad strolled across the stage to receive his diploma, Jean held 'replacement me' high up in the air. His serious face cracked, resulting in an attempt to retain his laughter as he continued his walk of achievement. My family made sure to include "me" in the photoshoot afterwards. At the very least, I was there to congratulate him in spirit.

To celebrate Mother's Day, we had a small cookout outside on our deck. Jean filled all of my pottery with artificial flowers in varying shades of blues and greens to match my navy rug plastered with bright lime and white flowers. Our deck overlooked a vast pasture field sprawling with the occasional cattle and spanned nearly the entire side of our home. Three old water maple trees shaded my oasis as the large creek flowed silently by in front of me. The oversized daybed filled with an abundance of plush pillows was by far my favorite place to curl up, read a book or just relax. The sun was peeking through the trees, a gentle breeze surrounded us as we enjoyed being together.

Still suffering from severe insomnia, along with a considerable amount of pain, I quickly became bored with the same routine in the house every day. On occasion, we would go on short drives along country roads, taking in the lush green leaves that now fully covered the tall trees. Joey put a smile on our faces watching the warm air slick his furry curls and floppy ears back as he hung his head outside the window. We would stop at local dairy bars to indulge in my go-to these days: a twist ice cream cone topped with cherry dip. It was nearly impossible for me to taste my food, therefore, anything other than my frozen treat would be heavily doused in A1 steak sauce, being the only thing I was able to taste.

Fun fact. I did not get the memo that my transplant could cause chemo-induced early menopause. I take back all of the times I made fun of my mother when she tore of her shirt in a rage to run outside in the cool air or press herself into the cold refrigerator. Out of nowhere, my entire body would feel as if I were boiling from the inside out. The back of my neck would be soaked with sweat. I would wake up in the middle of the night with my sheets covered in moisture. As if I didn't have enough issues I was dealing with at the moment, adding one more that I was unprepared for was deflating. I had just turned thirty-eight years old, was diagnosed with an incurable cancer and now a premature onset of menopause.

One dreary, rainy day, unsure if my emotions had gotten the best of me, or my newfound hormones introducing themselves, but I spent a solid six hours lying in bed bawling my eyes out. Shawn and Caleb alternated in and out of bed attempting to find some way of comforting me. I am certain they knew it was unchartered territory which left them lost and helpless. I was inconsolable. This entire time I had tried to project positivity but I desperately wanted to feel better. I yearned for sleep, which in this instance, I had worn myself down so much that my body finally succumbed to rest.

Seemingly out of nowhere, considering I was not on any chemotherapy at the moment, my face became fully covered with a prickly red rash. Picture it: bald head, hundreds of tiny red dots. Desperate for a remedy, I made an appointment with my dermatologist, also named Megan. She was tall, slender with long dark hair and big blue eyes. Shortly after my initial diagnosis, I contacted her office to cancel the annual check-up I already had scheduled with her. This resulted in a return phone call. Megan had been my dermatologist for several years so, she too, was shocked to hear the news of my diagnosis. Over the last few months, she has kept a sticky note with my name on it hanging from her computer screen to remind her to check in on me from time to time. I was touched she took time out of her day to remember me on occasion. We spent most of the exam catching up and she suggested I resume my chemo rash medications which thankfully got it under control.

On day ninety-six, my nephew was scheduled to enter this world and I was determined that nobody was going to keep me from meeting him. I was only four days away from my one hundred, therefore, I deemed myself safe enough to travel to Columbus to await his arrival. The room was filled with family members from both sides eagerly awaiting his birth. When we were finally told we were allowed back, I had been the only one paying attention and quickly darted down the hallway. Although there was a pre-determined order of who got to hold him, I was the person who met this beautiful baby boy first. Today, proudly wearing a royal blue t-shirt that read "Best Auntie Ever" in white, I was granted the title of Auntie Annie. I fell in love with Grayson Douglas immediately, his big brown eyes with a full head of dark hair. From this moment forward, anything he asked of me would instantly be his.

My best friend was getting married this summer! Megan was originally supposed to tie the knot in early July, however, when she found out I wouldn't be able to be there, she changed the date. A few weeks prior, she and I sat around my kitchen table to create her bouquet out of sage eucalyptus leaves and cream sola wood flowers. Today was her big day but it was also my much anticipated one hundredth day. She had made sure to announce my achievement to her guests prior to my arrival. I wore a lilac lace dress that matched the most amazing ruffled heels, completed with a darker blonde wig that I had attempted to elevate with a few big curls. As I slid out of the car on to the small pebbles beneath me, flocks of wedding goers began congratulating me on making it through the last one hundred days. I was quickly ushered into the large brick farmhouse where I spotted her right away. Megan was picture perfect in soft ivory lace, her long dark hair curled to one side. "Happy One Hundred Days" she said. Through hugs and tear-filled eyes, I thanked her but reiterated this was her big day, not mine. To her selfless soul, there was plenty of room today for both moments. As I watched her walk down the aisle, I could hear my son playing Canon in D softly on the violin as he sat underneath a nearby oak tree. I was beaming with so much love and excitement as my gorgeous friend began the rest of her life that day.

There had been several times I was ready to give up over the last few months. Although I had been warned, I did not anticipate just how difficult transplant, then recovery, would be. It definitely hasn't been easy, but I made it. One hundred days post-transplant. There wasn't a big celebration. Very few people understood the magnitude of this day. But that evening, as I stood barefoot in the soft grass of my backyard, I held up a sign that read "LouStrong – 100 Days" and snapped a photo, never wanting to forget this moment.

My last milestone: completed.

22
Life Without Milestones

Over the next couple of weeks, with a lot of help from my bestie, I planned a surprise sixtieth birthday party for my mom. Her brother came down from Pennsylvania and whisked her away for a couple hours to distract her. With the assistance of friends and family, their large pole barn was transformed to a peach floral wonderland full of photographs of her life thus far. Antique white doors topped with enormous coral and teal paper flowers lined the side of the barn, perfect for a photo backdrop. Jean was blown away when she returned to see the room filled with all her loved ones who were there to celebrate her. The icing on the cake was my brother, his wife and her new grandson had made the trip down as well. Caleb had the idea for us to record the song, We're Going to Be Friends, originally by the White Stripes, with an accompanying video for them, as it had been an important song to Chad as he was becoming a new dad. We made changes to some of the lyrics to make it more personal. Jean, Al, Caleb, Doug, Shawn & I were each given a single verse then all came together at the end. Caleb provided the music, using both guitar as well as a beautiful violin solo. The completed video was presented to the new parents at the party, resulting in tears of happiness. *Sissy's here to hold your hand. Tonight I'll dream while I'm in bed when silly thoughts run through my head, I can tell that we are gonna be friends....*

Summer was coming to an end. We moved Caleb into his new apartment near campus in Akron and though excited for his new chapter, I would again have to come to terms with not being able to see him every day. I missed my child so much already.

My bald head was now covered in a soft peach fuzz. I had been told that my wavy blonde hair would return darker, thicker and curlier. What I did not expect was the dark chocolate brown I saw when I looked in the mirror. I also noticed a stripe shortly above my left ear of smooth skin that apparently had always been there but never noticeable because of the hair covering it. Let me just tell you: new hair follicles poking through the skin is painful! It feels like there are hundreds of razor sharp needles pricking me all at once. I want to tear at my scalp to relieve the discomfort, however, that just makes it worse.

Once again, it was time to fill my body with a plethora of chemicals. I began replenishing my childhood vaccines with my first round of five shots. The high dose steroid, Dex, was added to my bone strengthener this time, in the hopes it may reduce the associated pain. I was prescribed two low dose hormone medications to combat the menopause side effects. Between the steroids and the hormones, my emotions were a mess. I felt a sense of déjà vu the night I began taking the Revlimid again. I stared down the clear plastic cup that held the blue and white pill that would both save my life and destroy it. Once I had cleared my one hundred days, I began a lower dose, ten instead of twenty-five, as maintenance therapy. There would be no breaks, no weeks off every month for my body to recover. Every. Single. Day. The side effects returned immediately. My face, chest and thighs were once again covered with bright red dots. The fatigue, frequent trips to the bathroom, constant joint pain, along with seemingly new issues were a permanent reminder of my condition. I found myself constantly itching my head, not due to dry scalp, but another side effect that released an incontrollable itch internally.

This was it. I had now officially begun my "new normal" and I hated it. I would remain on this chemotherapy for life, until a cure was discovered or a change was needed when my body becomes resistant to it. Depression soon took over which worried those closest to me. I would utter my usual "I'm Fine" fully aware I wasn't fooling anyone. Up until this point, I had remained positive so that my loved ones felt better. I wanted to ease any burden or worry they were dealing with as, they too, had to go through this diagnosis. But it wasn't fair to them to have to suffer along with me. It wasn't fair their lives had to change too. If I am being honest, it wasn't fair they had to watch me in this condition either.

My round the clock babysitting needs had come to an end. While I was happy to resume some tasks on my own again, it also meant I was now alone with my thoughts. I was struggling, emotionally, mentally and physically. I missed the ability to do normal activities. I yearned to return to work but some days I was unable to get out of bed, let alone drag myself to my job. It was also during this time I would learn a hard lesson of who would stand by me in my darkest hours. My heart was broken on more than one occasion by some of those closest to me. The betrayal weighed heavy on my soul. In the period of my life when I was grasping at straws more than any other time I can recall, desperately needing unconditional love, there were those who failed me. In the end, things would all work out and I would move past it, but it is a time in my life I would much rather forget.

Since the beginning of my diagnosis, I had set milestones to complete. Four cycles of chemo, pre-testing, harvest, transplant and one hundred days, each of which gave me something to look forward to completing. I had reached the end. There were no more goals. Nothing to look forward to in the future. Only a "new normal" of daily chemo pills, constant fatigue among other side effects and doing my best to stay away from illnesses. I do well with a plan, but as of now, I no longer have one. There were no more milestones to complete. My future appeared empty.

It was a dark road for a few weeks, one that was difficult for my family to endure. I can't say that I still don't have the same feelings sometimes, but on most days, I have learned to channel them in to more positive thoughts or activities. I plastered the dresser beside my bed with sticky notes that read quotes such as "Beautiful girl, you can do hard things" and "Straighten your crown." I began keeping a gratitude journal, writing down something I was grateful for that day. Sometimes it was as simple as the sky was blue, other days I found difficult to write anything at all but forced myself to do so. I resumed baking and crafting when I felt up to the task.

Much to my surprise, the following month I was given permission to return to Destin for another September trip! I would be required to wear a mask on the airplane, avoid crowded spaces and stay out of public pools. I was given a break from the Revlimid while I was there in order to provide more energy as well as a bump in my fragile immune system. Fishing boats were forbidden due to the risk of fracturing my brittle bones. I didn't care. I would handle any restrictions I was given if that meant I was allowed to return to what felt like our second home.

In what would become quite common for me any time I attempted to do something big, an issue would arise. A few days before our scheduled trip, I became so sick that I couldn't overcome the fever. This resulted in exams, bloodwork and imaging. Fully aware of how excited I was for this getaway, my doctor prescribed several medications with the hope I would feel better within a few days. Our departure date came, and though somewhat better, I was still feeling rough. I tried desperately to hide it with the assurance "I'm Fine" with a look that insinuated not to try to stop me. Jean and Al accompanied us down and we would pick up Caleb with his girlfriend, Alex, later that day. After a quick ninety-minute direct flight, I was greeted with the warm, familiar Florida air the moment I walked out the sliding airport door. We had cancelled our annual April trip so I had been anxiously awaiting our return. I threw my hands up in the air letting the sun beam down over my pale face as I took it all in.

We always stayed in the same room in the Sunset Suites of the Emerald Grande which stood tall across the bridge welcoming everyone to Destin. Our room resembled a large apartment that included a full-size kitchen, massive dining table and a living room large enough for us all to enjoy together. We had grown comfortable in this space over the years. Most of our time was spent out on the balcony closed off by ornate iron posts, overlooking the clear blue harbor by the East Pass, bustling with boats of varying sizes, jet skis and tourist excursions. Crab Island could be seen on our right, a sandbar with breathtaking crystal clear teal shallow water where pontoons gathered around for the day. Hundreds of people could be seen relaxing on inflatable floaties, rolling by on paddleboards and enjoying a snack from one of the vendor boats. Our room sat atop the Harborwalk Village, an extensive concrete boardwalk that ran along the harbor, consisting of shops, restaurants, the marina and nightlife.

To celebrate the occasion, I etched *LouStrong* next to a butterfly in the sand. As the sun set that evening, the sky a pale pink merging into gold, I sat silently alongside my artwork staring off in to the emerald waves crashing against the beach. I could listen to this sound all day, the gentle breeze sweeping by my face as I closed my eyes. I was wearing my grey and burgundy butterfly shirt, denim shorts, my hair now a chestnut brown buzz cut complete with a side stripe. In this moment, I was content. I wasn't thinking about my life with cancer.

The week was perfect. We spent time relaxing on the powder white sands that covered the beaches, occasionally cooling off in the crystal waters. My favorite days existed at Crab Island, enjoying time together as a family. We rotated listening to music on the pontoon, floating around on rainbow striped inflatable chairs connected by rope in order to keep us from disappearing from one another and teasing Jean as she waded over to acquire her brown bag of piping hot french fries. Watching her stroll across the waist deep water, holding her reward high above her head to prevent them from getting wet, was always a sight to see. Everyone was laughing, relaxing and having an amazing time. As I sat on the boat, wearing a lime green rash guard that covered my dark teal flowered bikini, protected by a large white sunhat with a turquoise scarf around it, I quietly examined my family. These people were essential in getting me where I was today. Without them, I wouldn't have had the strength and positivity to get through the last several months. My heart beamed with love for them as I took in the smiles on all their faces. They needed this vacation just as much as I did. The role of caretaker is equally exhausting. When the song, "Somewhere on a Beach", by Dierks Bentley, came through the speakers, my husband pulled me in to the warm water and wrapped his arms around me. We began singing the song, dancing in the water as if nobody was watching, finding myself giggling throughout the serenade. I never wanted this moment to end, to return home to reality.

We spent our final day with lunch at Boshamps on the harbor, a must do for every trip, where we indulged in hot, melty, pimento cheese dip topped with bacon jam, fried grouper sandwiches with spicy pickles and fresh cut french fries dipped in house made ranch. This was by far, the best restaurant on the Emerald Coast. That evening, we strolled along the Harborwalk, admiring the fish being brought in from the days catch. We enjoyed frozen drinks in both pineapples and baby watermelons as we took in the live music. The air was cool yet humid, the perfect weather to end our trip. After picking up yet another soft aqua blue sweatshirt that read DESTIN across the chest, we headed back to our room to finish packing for our early morning flight. My body was exhausted, however, over the entire week, it had only been necessary for me to stay in bed and re-cooperate just one day. I considered that a success. It was all worth every minute.

As the plane descended down the runway, taking off in to the clouds, I took in my surroundings, a vast area of blue waters below me. I already missed it. The mask covering my face reminded me it was time to return to reality, to resume my chemo pills, back to my new normal.

23
Too Much

As the leaves began to change to shades of gold and orange, we lost Shawn's Aunt Janet. From the first time I met her, we had an instant connection. We both shared a love for cooking and crafting and she reminded me so much of her sister, Shawn's mom, Carol. My diagnosis broke Janet's heart and she would often send me beautiful handmade cards wishing me the best. She would always sign them "I love you very much". Unable to say our final goodbyes in the hospital due to my condition, her son granted us a Facetime with her. In true fashion, she was more concerned about my health than hers. Her passing broke my heart and we miss her dearly.

I had kept my distance from my grandmother, who I call Mammy, over the last few months. I knew she wouldn't understand my diagnosis, nor my new hair, and I didn't want to upset her. When my Pappy passed away, she developed dementia. They had been married sixty-six years and she was lost without him. My Pappy was a hardworking, gentle man with thick glasses, baby blue eyes, a full head of snow white hair with a well fed belly, courtesy of my Mammy. He called me his *Annie Okey, Okey Pokey.* His last words to me, as I laid with him watching a black and white western on the nursing home television, were to take care of my Mammy and that he loved me. I miss him beyond measure. Losing a grandparent is a loss that I will never fully recover from. During our weekly phone calls, she would inquire as to why I hadn't come to see her, to which I explained I had been sick. Coincidentally, she had a bone density test the same date and location as my annual gynecological exam and mammogram, therefore, we went to our appointments together. I had forgotten to wear my wig to pick her up, to which she immediately expressed her displeasure with my new "hair cut". Mammy was a tall, thin woman with perfectly placed salt and pepper curls, clear glasses and a large black purse she guarded with her life. She was ornery, went through two boxes of snack cakes a week and loved bologna sandwiches. Her answer to how she was doing was always "fine as frog's hair". After our imaging was complete, she sat in the corner of my room, next to my clothes as I sat on the exam table. In true form, my goofy grandmother, while giggling, flicked my underwear at me from across the room, just as my doctor walked in. My doctor is a petite woman with sleek dark hair, caramel skin and a gentle smile. Another amazing addition to my medical team. She introduced herself to Mammy, who responded to her by telling her she didn't like my hair since I cut it short and dark, stating that I now looked like a boy. My doctor responded that she thought I looked beautiful. Nevertheless, I enjoyed spending the day with my Mammy. She only remembered a handful of family members now and I was still one of them. I was grateful for that, as watching someone you love forget everything they knew in life, is heartbreaking. I took no offense to her remarks, fully aware she was unable to understand my condition.

My mammogram showed a few spots of concern, which prompted a follow up ultrasound. I knew when the radiologist came in the room after the nurse had completed the imaging it was not good news. He gently explained to me that there were two areas he believed were Stage Zero breast cancer, suggesting a biopsy to confirm. I sat there listening as if I was having an out of body experience. This could not be happening. I knew the Revlimid could cause secondary cancers, including breast cancer, but I had only been taking it for a year. My appointment now a blur, I shut the door to my car and began ugly crying in the parking lot. How was I going to tell Shawn? My Mom? Could they go through all of this again? Did I have the strength to endure it?

I had my monthly appointment at Strecker already scheduled for the next day. When Dr. Cawley walked in the room she began with "I'm so sorry". She continued by telling me that I should be angry, have a good cry, but, although she didn't want me to go through all of this again, she was not worried. The treatment may suck for a while but this stage of breast cancer was not life threatening. Tears streamed down my face throughout the entire appointment as she drew detailed pictures for me to understand. As we left, though deflated, I felt more at ease with my newest diagnosis.

One week later, I was lying on a cold, sterile table, back aching, my arm extended awkwardly down through a hole, a large lidocaine needle being inserted into my breast. What I thought would be a quick procedure, turned extensive when the numbing needle moved the mass to a different area that the doctor could not seem to locate. The feeling of a biopsy needle shoving in and out of my body over and over again on a fishing expedition to find its desired target was anything but comfortable. My arm had fallen asleep, the numbing wore off, requiring a second dose, and I had grown annoyed. After what seemed like hours, the biopsy was finally achieved.

Shawn had to work, therefore, Caleb had the job of taking care of me for the remainder of the day. It was rather strange having my son switch out my ice packs from the freezer every fifteen minutes as required, but Warden Jr. was insistent I stay in bed, and I obliged, sleeping away the remainder of the day. The next morning, Dr. Cawley called me, ecstatic that the biopsies came back as benign! I did not have breast cancer. A huge rush of relief came over me. I immediately called Shawn, who was in the woods, deer trolling with a friend, to ease his mind with this good news. He fell to the ground, releasing all of the fear he had been holding inside, allowing it to flow out of him onto the forest floor.

When it rains, it pours. Shawn had recently suffered a few nerve issues which finally landed him at the neurologist's office. It was determined he would need neck surgery immediately. Megan accompanied us to Columbus to assist in the drive home as well as moral support. The last procedure my husband had done under anesthesia resulted in complications, so we were both concerned about the surgery. One year after my initial stay in the hospital, it was now my turn to be strong for my spouse. Holding his hand, I kissed him on the forehead and promised him I would see him soon. A crazy worrier by nature, my eyes were glued to the screen in the waiting room, impatiently awaiting the icons to change from surgery to recovery. I longed to be with him in the operating room holding his hand. I was grateful Megan was there to keep me distracted with friendly conversations. My mind was put to ease when the doctor came out to assure me of the success of the surgery. When my husband was finally wheeled in to the recovery room, he grabbed at his chest, desperately searching for a glowing plate, believing he was, in fact, Iron Man. It was quite amusing and something we have never let him forget. Shawn often suffers from migraines and the surgery had provoked a severe one. Unable to get the pain under control with the offered pain medications, he was suffering in agony. I stayed loyal by his bed, holding his hand while gently rubbing his forehead. At midnight, Megan finally convinced me it was time to check in to the hotel next door. We collapsed into our beds, which held the softest, most comfortable mattress and pillow I have slept in to date. Megan and I still reminisce about the comfort of those beds. It was like being engulfed in a fluffy cloud. It was New Year's Eve when I awoke, still concerned for my husband, wondering if his head was still throbbing. Shortly thereafter, he called me, letting me know he was ready to go home and needed better coffee. We walked in his room to a new man from the previous evening. Shawn is most likely the worst patient in the world. Ignoring the fact that he was told not to get out of bed on his own, he had roamed the halls throughout the night by himself, only to be warned and ushered back to bed each time. I am surprised they didn't give up and restrain him to the bed. Much to his nurse's displeasure, Shawn had also taken his own medication that he found in his duffel bag. Having decided he was ready to go home, not wanting to wait for the discharge papers, he had just begun to take out his IV when we arrived to stop him. Worst. Patient. Ever. Although he had to wear a neck brace for a few weeks, his recovery was fairly quick, his scar nearly unrecognizable and his previous symptoms mostly healed.

The last three months had been filled with a wide array of emotions. We suffered a death in the family, another cancer scare, as well as a major surgery. I was ready to leave this year behind to start anew.

24
The Pandemic

It was advised that I stay indoors during my first post-transplant winter season and I did so accordingly. On the first day of February, we finally went out for a date night, consisting of dinner and a movie. Of course, the next day I woke up sick. Apparently, along with losing all of my childhood vaccines, I also lost all immunities to illnesses and allergies I had built up over the years. It would take me several weeks to overcome and feel better. And then, the beginning of the Covid pandemic frightened the world. Just when I thought I was able to live life somewhat normally again, I was put into quarantine, unable to leave the house. So many people were dying from this unknown disease, especially those who were immunocompromised, like myself. The world was filled with uncertainty and I was not willing to take the risk.

My tribe immediately sprung into action. For years, I have sleep-walked in the middle of the night, eating Swiss Rolls out of the refrigerator. Several of my friends began porch dropping boxes of the chocolate cakes with cream filling, ensuring I would not run out of them. Others dropped off grocery staples, such as milk and bread, so we didn't have exposure at the store. It was heartwarming to know, that even a year after my initial diagnosis, my friends and family stepped up to make my life easier.

As time went on and people were passing away by the thousands, my time in quarantine was filled with fear, boredom and depression, with no end in sight. The world had nearly shut down. I missed human interaction. Thus, the beginning of the door visits. My family and friends began stopping by to sit outside my front door to spend time with me. Hanging on my glass screen door was a wreath of sage green hydrangeas, white lilies and small chocolate flowers that I had created from my leftover wedding flowers. It became a funny tradition that everyone who came over would take a photo of their faces smiling at me through the wreath. I looked forward to my chats through the door brightening my day. Mom would stop by to see me almost daily, parking herself in a chair on the other side of the glass.

Digital communication became imperative. Weekly zoom calls with Mom, Chad and Caleb became the highlight of my week. They were always full of laughter and witty conversation that instantly brightened my spirits. Megan began Facetiming me whenever she went to the grocery store as well as an occasional driving around in her car to "get me out". It soon became a fun excursion around town.

The day of my stem cell transplant is also known as a re-birthday, therefore, becoming a day to celebrate every year. Shawn refers to April 17th as the day that gave him his wife back. My first re-birthday was spent in quarantine. To commemorate this occasion, I decided to dye my short dark hair, now sprouting a very wild cowlick, a burgundy color, put on a new Multiple Myeloma shirt and do a little photo shoot at home. Everyone loved the new look, noting how much it brightened my green eyes. This would begin a new tradition of changing my hair color to my cancer ribbon color on every re-birthday. My mom had secretly arranged a card shower for me, resulting in a multitude of gorgeous cards congratulating me on my achievement. I am a firm believer in the simple things in life and these cards warmed my heart more than anyone could imagine. I was truly blessed to have such an amazing support system.

Caleb drove down to surprise me for Mother's Day with a cookout on our deck. Every part of my being wanted to embrace my child without letting go, but I was stuck behind the screen french doors, still quarantined in the beginning of the pandemic. Caleb would graduate from college this week, silently, as they had cancelled the commencement. He would be receiving his Bachelor's Degree in Social Work in only two years, due to the fact he achieved his Associates Degree while still in high school. Caleb had also been accepted into a Masters program in Cleveland that he would be beginning online classes in a few weeks. This Momma was beyond proud of all my son's accomplishments and couldn't wait to see the great things I knew he would do with his life. I had been collecting cards and gifts from loved ones congratulating him that I had planned to mail out the following week. Now that he was here, I was able to watch him open his surprises as he sat on the lime green daybed overflowing with royal blue pillows. I wanted him to come inside and stay the night in his bedroom. I needed a hug from my child. These luxuries were unattainable due to the possibility I could contract Covid. I forced a smile as I said goodbye to him that day, but tears ran down my face as I watched his car drive off into the distance. I resented all this pandemic was taking from me.

It had been months since I had been out of the house for anything other than doctor appointments. As Covid guidelines and restrictions began to ease slightly, I was able to visit with Mom or Megan during deck dates, outside, remaining six feet apart. I would take these as a win and soak up every minute of them. My doctors approved a trip to Hocking Hills for our ten year anniversary in July, which was located about ninety minutes from our house. It was a state forest with magnificent rock formations and several hiking trails with waterfalls. We rented a quaint cabin surrounded by tall green trees and a vast pond. Kindred Spirits is one of my all-time favorite restaurants nestled in an old log cabin. We ordered our usual, a thick grilled pork chop with chipotle maple glaze, mouthwatering wild rice and spring salad topped with shaved parmesan, this time as a carry out meal to take back to our cabin to enjoy a romantic meal just for two. The remainder of the evening was spent in the hot tub, where my husband would invent a new hip hop dance move, one I will always remember, then relaxing in adirondack chairs around a fire. As amazing as the day was, in typical fashion, I became severely dehydrated, not taking into account the wine I had that evening, resulting in us leaving our trip a day early to spend the next day at the Cancer Center to receive an infusion instead. I was deflated. Angry at myself for ruining our weekend. Shawn reassured me that we had an amazing day together so I was being ridiculous. No matter what he said, I was determined that I had ruined it for us both.

During one of my Covid appointments, I wore a lilac shirt that read *It's Fine, I'm Fine, Everything is* Fine in teal. Marcia, my nurse practitioner, walked into the room, immediately shaking her head at me when she noticed my statement. I pride myself for my bubbly personality and thought it would provide us both a good laugh. Multiple Myeloma patients are required to get imaging known as a Skeletal Survey annually in search for lesions. We knew that it would show that I would need another back surgery at some point, but we were unprepared for the other gut punch it would reveal. When I was first diagnosed, I had bone lesions on my spine, hip, ribs, sternum and collarbone. We were now told that I had a new lesion on my femur. I felt like I couldn't breathe. I was only a little over a year post transplant. It was too soon. I wasn't ready to go through all of this again. I couldn't do it again. My doctor had hoped I would get a longer response from the transplant, but reminded me that my kappa light chains had also been increasing over the last couple of months. She scheduled additional imaging for me as the torture of the waiting game began. Our minds were constantly fearing the worst, chests remaining tight, each trying to force strength for the other. I was terrified. I wanted to hide under a blanket away from everything and everyone and pretend it wasn't real.

That same week, I had an appointment at the James with my new specialist, Dr. Bumma. I didn't have anything against my former doctor, however, I just wasn't connecting with him on a personal level. I instantly cliqued with my new doctor. He had darker skin with black curly hair slicked back in a low pony tail, charcoal glasses and scruffy facial hair on the verge of turning grey. Shawn was instructed to stay in the car but he attended via Facetime. My new doctor was patient in listening to all of my concerns, responding with in depth, informative answers. He instructed me to think of my bones as wood and my lesions as termites. You can take care of the termites but the damage is still there causing my bones to be brittle. After reviewing my imaging, he was confident I did not have a new lesion, but rather something known as a venous lake, which was a small cluster of blood vessels. The last several days have been devastating for all of us believing my cancer had become more aggressive so soon. We all lived in fear and on edge filled with anxiety. I was now overcome with a rush of relief, followed by frustration that I even had to deal with all of those emotions that ended up being unnecessary. I explained that I was having a hard time dealing with my 'new normal' and the pandemic restrictions making it even more difficult. He looked me straight in the eye with such sincerity, reminded me that I have an incurable cancer that will present itself in many phases, but his goal was to keep me alive until there is a cure. My kappa light chains have continued to rise, but thankfully not enough yet to increase my chemo dosage. I left the appointment feeling confident I had made the right decision in changing specialists, knowing he was the right fit for me.

We had to cancel yet another trip to Destin this past spring, so I was surprised and overjoyed when my doctors allowed me to go in the fall. Jean and Al would be required to Covid test, then quarantine a few days before the trip. We would all be required to wear masks, both on the plane, as well as anywhere we would go in Florida. To celebrate the occasion, I had a LouStrong butterfly constructed in the sand, which was fascinating to watch come to life. It stood as tall as I was sitting beside it. Along with burgundy hair, a sand sculpture would now become a yearly tradition. Unfortunately, this trip ended up being cut short due to an incoming hurricane near the area. Determined that I was not going to let my first week off chemo in a year go to waste, we spent the remainder of the week back at Hocking Hills, where I would even successfully navigate the quarter mile handicap accessible path to Ash Cave. I had forgotten just how normal I could feel again when I didn't have a constant daily chemo pill dragging my body down.

When we returned from our getaway, I hid in the shower, succumbing to a good cry, again not wanting to resume the blue and white pill. Shawn walked in the bathroom, catching me in the act. In that moment, he opened the door, stepped into the shower, fully clothed, just to hold me. Another one of the many reasons I love this passionate, patient, unselfish man of mine. Anyone who knows me can attest to the fact that nobody is allowed to touch me when I am trying to remain strong but ready to break inside. A simple hug will surely bring on a waterfall of tears. Per usual, they would just be assured that I was fine. My husband's embrace is strong yet gentle, much like he himself is, and in that raw moment, I collapsed in to his chest, letting go of all self control. After what seemed like hours, but was surely only minutes, I dried myself off, wiped my sore red eyes and slid my nemesis down my throat. I would have to learn to enjoy the chemo breaks when I was allowed to have them while accepting the fact that I needed those pills to live a longer life. This is something I am not sure if I will ever fully accept but I cannot change.

I love all genres of music from country to hip hop to songs of the eighties. My favorite playlist is simply titled *Inspiration*. Shawn often questions why I listen to such songs that often result in a few tears, but to me, it is full of words that I relate to. The tears aren't necessarily from sadness, but more of a deep understanding or a reminder. "Amazing Grace" will always remind me of my Bubba singing it from the top of her lungs like nobody was watching. "In The Garden" is the song my mother calmed us with as children. One of my favorites, "I'm Standing with You", by Chrissy Metz, makes my heart swell thinking of my relationship with my husband.

> *When you're hurting, I want you to know*
> *That you'll never have to hurt alone*
> *When you think that all the odds*
> *are all against you*
> *And you just feel giving up, well I won't let you.*
> *We all got times when we can't be strong*
> *When it feels like all hope is gone*
> *But I'm right here, right here to lean on*
> *I'll always be strong for you*
> *Through whatever you go through*
> *I'm standing with you*

I love this song because I know every word of it is true for my husband. He is my strength when I am weak. He truly sees me no differently than before I had cancer, protects me at all cost and loves me so fiercely and genuinely. Music has always held a special place in both our hearts. Some music is meaningful, others remind us of our pontoon playlist, while some take us back to all the concerts we have attended in the past.

We made a commitment to have an outdoor date night once a week, picking up our dinner to go, enjoying different locations by the river or in a park. My husband has always been a true romantic and is known to drop everything to embrace me for a dance in the kitchen. He looks me straight in the eye while serenading me with whatever song reminds him of me in this moment. I melt right into him, thankful we can disappear in each other's arms to escape for a short moment. Most of my fondest memories surround the kitchen, these dances, cooking with my child, baking cookies with my Bubba and countless other memories. I am grateful for all the memories made in our tiny home.

Our date nights would also include picnics on our deck, which had recently been extended by Shawn and my dad. They completed the addition just in time for our new hot tub to be delivered, right as the leaves were beginning to change. The first time I slid into the heated bubbling water I felt an immediate sense of relief. My sore muscles pelted by jets, I took in the view off our deck overlooking the vast pasture field, flowing creek and black cattle in the distance. I was grateful to be a country girl.

My husband's daily routine has always been to tell me he loves me while reminding me that I am beautiful, both before and after cancer. When I looked in the mirror, I no longer recognized myself, sunken face, tiny frame and out of control dark brown hair that most certainly resembled a mullet. As I stood in front of my reflection one morning, Shawn put his hands around my face, looked me straight in my eyes and said "I see you". Though he may, I still did not. My hair was finally at a length where I was able to add a few blonde highlights along with a much-needed trim. I knew my hair needed shaped properly but still held my breath as I watched the tiny pieces fall to the ground. I had worked for over a year to grow the short amount of hair I had achieved thus far. It was difficult to watch any of it be cut away. Closer to my original color, I felt more like myself for the first time in a long time.

In December, my absolute neutrophil count, also known as ANC, a type of white blood cell that fights infections, dropped to below 1.0. Due to this, as well as a decline in other lab results, my doctors felt it was best to cut my Revlimid dosage in half. I was hopeful that the lower amount of chemo would allow my body to feel better on a daily basis, however, I was also incredibly nervous about the change. My kappa had been slowly climbing over the last several months. Would the new dosage be enough to control my cancer cells? Nevertheless, I began my new regimen right away.

One of the hardest things to deal with during the pandemic, especially for an immunocompromised person, was not being able to spend time with family. The holidays were approaching and we were unsure of how they would be celebrated this year. Luckily, there is an enormous pole barn on the farm, complete with a kitchen that held several long, spaced apart, tables. Because nobody was taking the risk of spending the night with each other, Shawn and I spent Christmas morning with just the two of us. It would be the first year Caleb was not here to open his presents after the sun came up. The mother in me missed that tradition desperately. Fire crackling, carols playing in the background, the smell of hot coffee filling the air, Shawn and I took turns sharing gifts and laughing at Joey sticking his nose in his new bag of treats. Later that morning, we all sent photos of our negative Covid tests in our group text. With everyone passing, the family all set out to arrive for dinner. Jean had decorated the barn with a new Christmas tree set in front of a barnwood backdrop. White ceramic ornaments with each of our names in black scroll hung from ribbon on pine green garland. Along with making ornaments this year to surpass some of my boredom time, I was excited to create fun ways to wrap this years' gifts. Boxes were stacked on top of each other, wrapped in different colors and adorned with final touches. A snowman was mostly white, a black hat with green holly, cardstock orange nose and buttons with a scarlet and black scarf. A red Santa with a cotton beard and his accompanying chartreuse elf with red and white striped bottom stood three feet tall. We had taken the precaution of wearing masks, only removing them for a family photo, all matching in coordinating red, green or white buffalo check thermal pants. It wasn't the family Christmas we were accustomed to, but we were still able, in all of the uncertainty, to spend time together. That is what mattered the most. That evening, as I did every year, I carefully turned the crank to play Silent Night on my grandmother's white ceramic tree, light shining through the bright blue bulbs and birds. It was the month of December, five years ago now, that I had lost my Bubba and my heart still ached for her. I sat there in the dark reminiscing until the music stopped playing, then headed off to bed praying that she just might visit me in my dreams.

As this crazy year was coming to an end, I had decided to finally give in to trying medical marijuana. Although I had the drugs in my possession for a couple of months, I was nervous about trying them. I did not want to be in a state of mind where I could not remember things or be out of control. I was still dealing with the grief of my initial diagnosis. I was so intoxicated during my stay at

Riverside that I had not gone through the feelings that accompanied being diagnosed with cancer. My family had to sit there, day after day, waiting on results and struggling internally. I was not part of that experience, one that they prefer not to relive, but something I felt like I was missing. I was not in control of myself during that time, which was something that I was scared of feeling again. The staff at the dispensary assured me that there were different strands of marijuana, to which I informed them I did not want to feel out of my mind. I was given a sleep weed oil as well as a gummy promised to relieve body pain. Nervously, I placed a quarter of the recommended dose of oil underneath my tongue. Within ten minutes, I was giggling, shortly followed by a few hours of deep sleep.

25
Caregivers

I often think about the role of a caregiver, along with all of the responsibilities attached to it. One day out of the blue, their whole world is interrupted, forcing them in to a new title. When I was diagnosed, my husband and my mother were both shoved in to this new role. Fully aware that some people weren't fortunate enough to have a family caregiver, I have always felt beyond grateful that I did. However, with this, came an overwhelming amount of guilt for the lives they were putting on hold. Not only were they coming to terms with my diagnosis, they also had to force themselves to hold back their own emotions in order to project strength. They were giving up their daily lives to take care of me which, in my mind, was not fair to them. I was disrupting all they have ever known forcing them to change their lifestyles. They weren't given a manual to help guide them but they were fully invested in their new roles.

Shawn has always had to endure the brunt of it all. He is the one who is forced to watch all that I go through, mentally, emotionally, physically, around the clock, every single day. My husband is the most patient, compassionate, protective person I have ever known. To most of the outside world, Shawn is strong, stubborn and obsessed with telling deer stories and dad jokes, but at home, he is really just a big teddy bear.

My husband and I had a wonderful marriage prior to my diagnosis; however, we have grown closer on an even deeper level. I think it is indicative of our relationship to spend years together in isolation due to cancer and then the pandemic, only to love each other even more. We rarely argue, and when we do, it somehow usually ends up with us laughing at one another. Shawn has the best laughter, bent over to his side, belly jiggling, tears in the corner of his eyes. We both find ourselves easily amused quite often. Our relationship began by spending hours in deep conversations and I think we have maintained that throughout our marriage. We constantly find ourselves in dialogues from the simplest to the deepest of topics. We enjoy spending time with each other in the smallest of things, such as sitting outside with a hot cup of coffee or driving in the country in pursuit of wildlife. Though we continue to do all of those things together, our dynamic of husband and wife is now coupled with caretaker and patient.

A caretaker is not only forced to take over all of the daily household chores, but more importantly, become a round the clock nurse. Shawn was given the daily task of shuffling through the pharmacy, overflowing with orange and white plastic bottles that now resided in one of our bathroom drawers, in order to fill my colorful pill boxes every week, as well as offer me all of the in between medications. I needed him to help me in and out of bed, to take a shower or make it to the car. He fed me on occasion when my hands were too shaky and calmed me down when I became mortified over it. These are just a few examples of my daily routine that I now required assistance with. Over time, I would be able to do certain things on my own again but there are still occasions I need his physical assistance. Stubborn sometimes to a fault, I have been known to frustrate him attempting to do things on my own, fully aware that I should not. It is often deflating not being able to do things on your own. I have always been fiercely independent, therefore, being told I could not complete a task wasn't acceptable.

The physical role of a caretaker eventually becomes routine, but the persistent mental and emotional toll it takes must be excruciating at times. Shawn lives in a constant state of worry for my condition, the dreaded waiting for test results and knowing how I am feeling by one look at my eyes while unable to make it better. He is always taking precautions at work or when we go out, terrified he may make me sick. My husband feels like he needs to always be the strong force in our relationship, though, at the same time, constantly reminding me that it is I who am the strongest one, not realizing we both hold that trait. For a long time, he refused to leave me for anything other than his job, even though I was continually pushing him to do something for himself. I am grateful for his work family, which realistically I should call *our* work family, because not only do they support him, but they have also been wonderful to me. It was hard for him to be around friends for a while, even keeping him away from one in particular because every time they spoke, he would break down. At one point, I even went behind his back, asking his friends to pressure him to go out and do things with them. Eventually, he began golfing and hunting again in small doses. I am fully aware just how much I mean to him, but he needed that time away from me, time to release and recharge doing something just for himself.

Though we express our urge to make life easier for our loved ones in different ways, it is a trait I inherited from my mother. She did not have the best upbringing which left her with a constant need to please people and to take care of them. When I became ill, her entire world stopped, switching her life's mission to taking care of her daughter. Nothing else mattered. She cancelled her vacations through all of my objections, missed out on outings with her friends, leaving her whole life to revolve around me. Her daily routine consisted of work, doting on me, housekeeping, sleep, repeat for nearly a year. Shawn was here with me the majority of the time that she was, however, Jean was adamant she needed to be here too. My mom needed to see for herself how I was doing, needed to cook and clean for us, knowing that next door would not be close enough for her, for every second away was a constant worry in her head.

I can't imagine watching my child battle cancer. One of the first questions I asked my doctor was if mine was hereditary. All I could think of was what if I passed this down to my child. Thankfully, Multiple Myeloma is not well known as a hereditary cancer. I am positive that my mom would take my place in an instant if she could. It is a mother's job to protect her children but this was out of her hands. The only thing she could control was taking care of me to make my life a little easier. I have watched her painfully use all her internal strength to hold back her tears. I have seen her face attempt to hide herself crumbling inside. I grew up with my mother as my role model for teaching me to be strong.

As time went by and my mom returned to her own home more often, she sometimes finds it easier to live in denial. Often times, the constant roller coaster of my cancer is too much for her to bear. She no longer has to see my daily struggles and I am good at putting on a brave face to deter her. She loathes when I tell her that I'm fine, knowing full well I am bending the truth at times. It is easier to pretend it isn't real sometimes just to get by. Having said that, she is always there for me without hesitation.

There isn't a doubt in my mind that there is nothing in this world either of them would not do for me. Shawn has been forced to maintain the brunt of the role of caretaker. He is the one who endures my everyday life of what others don't see. I made the mistake once of telling him he would be better off without me, citing it was not fair for him to take care of me day after day. He was furious, insisting we take care of each other and that a life without me wasn't a life worth living for him. We calmed one another, provided strength when the other was weak, made each other better people. He is my rock, my person, and I am certain that I wouldn't be where I am today without his love and support. He was put in my life for a reason.

My caretakers took their roles very seriously, which led them wanting to do everything for me. If I got up to fill my water bottle, one of them would grab it for me. When I moved laundry out of the washer to the dryer, the clothes were removed from my hands. They had become so accustomed to doing things for me they did not realize I needed to learn to do some things on my own again. I wanted them to see me beyond the tunnel vision that came with my cancer. I became desperate to experience some sort of normality from my previous life. It was extremely difficult for them to let go, wanting nothing more than to make my life easier. But I couldn't get better if I was constantly being told I was not allowed to do something. How could I push forward if I was constantly being held back? To be fair, I would often attempt to do one thing or another fully aware it was a bad idea, therefore, forcing me to compromise with them. Eventually, and very reluctantly, my caretakers and I found balance, allowing me to get back to doing small things when I felt able, but giving in to continuing to allow them to help me when warranted.

I imagine caretakers often feel isolated and alone as they provide a constant strength for their loved one. Their world is changed in an instant making it a challenge to balance their new role with their normal routines. I struggle knowing I am the cause of the upset in their lives. I will be forever grateful to my husband and my mother for all they gave up to take care of me. They will never see it as a burden but I will always carry the guilt for what they gave up and continue to endure.

26

Joey

I have had several dogs over the years but it was fate that brought Joey into our lives. Initially, Joey was supposed to be Caleb's dog, but it was quickly evident that he chose me as his person. Cavapoos are a cross between a Cavalier King Charles Spaniel and a Poodle. They are an intelligent, super cuddly, sweet breed. Our pup was a bit of a hopper when he was little, always providing us with a giggle from all the cuteness. He was eager to play toys and perfected a complete three sixty circle maneuver when he was awaiting the throw of his favorite purple squeaky bone. Although he enjoyed playing with his toys, Joey was most content snuggled up on my chest.

When I returned home from Riverside, he instantly knew something was wrong. He came running to me, but slid to a complete stop along the wood floors. He was still prancing, attempting to control the overwhelming urge to greet me with the usual slippery wet ear kisses. He had been away from us for ten days. From this day forward, Joey refused to leave my side, always at my right ankle following at my pace. When I slept, he nestled his warm body against mine. That first week, when Shawn came anywhere near me, Joey sat up to growl at him, not a mean snarl, but rather a playful one alerting Shawn that his new role was solely my protector. He followed along my every step as I learned to move with a walker. My physical therapist immediately thought by his behavior that he was a trained service dog.

After the first year, and as the pandemic took over the world, I was often alone, and like many others during this time, felt isolated. I had plenty of friends and family doing all they could to stay present in my life, but during this time, it just wasn't all I needed. Joey quickly became my life line. I needed this dog. He diverted my mind to focus on him rather than all the negative thoughts circling in my head. When I feel like wallowing in bed all day, he forces me to get up to take him outside. If I am hurt, he licks my wounds. When I cry, he licks my tears, forcing me to laugh. Sometimes, his cuddles are all I need to get through the day. All it takes is one look at his furry teddy bear appearance to smile. He tilts his head to one side listening to me talk to him which I am convinced is the most adorable thing ever.

As time went by, someone suggested to me that I have him trained as a service dog. I ended up contacting a locally owned training company run solely by veterans. I have the utmost respect for our military and at one point or another I have been affiliated with every branch. On our first meeting, I was advised that, though they would try to train him, Joey was older now so they were unsure if they would be successful. Well, Joey was a star student and six short weeks later, my pup was a certified Service Dog who took his job very seriously! Cavapoos are known to be a highly intelligent breed, loyal to their owners, and Joey took to his new tasks quickly and seriously. I still get an occasional message from his trainer noting something they came across in a guide citing Joey was the anomaly in the training world of older dogs. At that time, he had been trained for three tasks. He performs those no matter the situation, however, he is fully aware when we are out with his vest on that he has other rules to follow. If someone reaches out to pet him, he will step behind me, knowing he is working and isn't allowed to be doted upon. It is absolutely amazing to me how this sweet little pup of mine has learned how to take care of me in far more ways than emotional support.

I think it is often difficult for some to understand the bond one forms with their dog, especially in my situation. To me, Joey is not "just a dog". I am rarely without him. He is always by my side wherever I go. There are a couple rare situations where I am unable to take him with me due to personal preferences, where I have to make a choice to attend something, leaving him behind, or forego it. This has become one of my biggest struggles. Not only am I used to having him with me around the clock, but he has also become accustomed to never being alone. If I have to leave him, I know that he does not move from his position on the window seat, howling and whining until I return. It causes me an infinite amount of anxiety knowing what the separation is doing to both of us. I am torn with the choice of attending something, fighting through the torture, or simply not participating. Either decision breaks my heart. He is a part of me now. Joey is most certainly like my child. I need this adorable, caramel colored furry little pup full of curls with human eyes and cute floppy ears. He is my protector in his own way. I can't imagine my life without him. In many ways, he has saved me.

27

Moving Forward

I was turning forty this year along with Caleb turning the big twenty-one! We had all received our first dose of the Covid vaccine, therefore, decided to celebrate together in a log cabin in Hocking Hills. Our weekend home was massive and sat alone in the woods surrounded by trees that were just beginning to blossom with fresh spring leaves. Taking precautions, we all wore masks, being quite used to the routine by now. My birthday cake was swirled with teal and purple rosettes, *80's girl* sprawled across the front in yellow, coordinating rock candy and twirl pops stuck out the top where a sparkly glitter 'forty' candle burnt. Turquoise and lavender balloons covered the floor of the dining room, complete with giant silver balloons, boasting both of our new ages. The day could not have been more perfect. We had a family dinner at my favorite restaurant, Kindred Spirits, followed by a waffle cone filled with cherry ice cream. Our evening was spent surrounding the fireplace playing a myriad of board games. I had found a rainbow parachute much like those in elementary school gym class. We all sat in a circle, moving it up and down, as my young nephew ran under it over and over again, often chased by my furry little pup. Such a simple game that brought us all a bit of fun and an abundance of laughter.

A couple weeks later, I had reached my second re-birthday. Per new tradition, I colored my nearly shoulder length hair a bright red burgundy. After acquiring matching balloons, we went downtown by the river to take a few photos to mark the occasion. I climbed atop the fountain, careful not to fall in the water. Perched on top the sprouting water, wearing a shirt that read *Cancer Survivor* in my color, I grasped the balloons while Shawn captured the moment in front of the clear blue sky. Two years after transplant, life was not easy, my numbers were slowly creeping up, but I was thankful to be here celebrating this day again.

Mother's Day this year would again coincide with another graduation. Caleb had completed his Master's program in just twelve months. He would be moving further north to Cleveland. Because commencements were still under Covid restrictions, he would indulge us by adorning his black and green cap and gown with a gold sash. I stood beside my son proudly wearing my green Cleveland State Mom shirt. At only twenty-one years old, Caleb was ready to start his new life. I could not wait to see all of the amazing things he was going to accomplish.

As the world was beginning to return to some sort of normality, though still taking precautions, I slowly began venturing out. Doug would pick me up for an occasional hot dog lunch down by the river. I felt comfortable enough to go shopping from time to time, continuing to wear a mask. It was rejuvenating just to be out of the house, no longer stuck in a constant state of isolation.

I had registered to be part of the Muscles for Myeloma Walk in Columbus earlier in the year, which, much like everything else, was cancelled, becoming a virtual event. Dark green shirts that read *Cure in Five* on the front were mailed to us along with our race number badges. I spent the morning curling my wavy, now shoulder length, blonde highlighted hair. Shawn and I drove down the gravel driveway that leads to the farm, Joey in tow, where we walked a short distance until my muscles gave out. We were asked to post a photo of our participation on the group Facebook page. I chose my favorite of the day, Shawn and I arm in arm, he kissing my cheek as I looked back at the camera. Cancer was a part of me now. I had made the decision to embrace the community support that came along with that diagnosis rather than hide from it. Shortly thereafter, I would participate in my first Relay for Life event.

I had been asked to be part of an event called Living Beyond Cancer by doing a video interview to be shown that evening. I was incredibly nervous as I have never been comfortable with public speaking. Sitting in front of a stone wall in my LouStrong t-shirt, my hair straightened and tucked behind my ears, I began telling the story of my diagnosis. I shared the scrapbook album I had put together that included my journaling, scans of my reports, test results and imaging as well as photos of my ever-changing appearance. I went on to say that I was going to live every day the best that it could be and accept the days my body says 'not today'. I am still going to go to the beach every chance I get, even though it may take extra rest days that I never needed before, as well as taking every opportunity to visit a new place or do something that I love. Fighting back tears, voice crackling, I continued that at the end of the day, I have cancer, one that does not have a cure, but I am also a survivor and I choose to take that title over simply a cancer patient. I urged others to stay positive, focus on milestones and stock up on Pedialyte. I finished the interview with a plea to remember that you are far stronger than you ever thought you could be, have faith you will get through this and never give up. I stayed over to listen to a pastor recite his history, riddled with a family who nearly all battle cancer. It was inspiring to listen to his story. As I drove home that afternoon, although I was initially hesitant, I was grateful for the opportunity that my ordeal may help someone else in the future.

In April, we enjoyed another visit to Destin. Keeping up with the new tradition, we had another sand castle constructed to celebrate my second re-birthday. This one stood five feet tall, resembling a castle of faux bricks and steps galore. Small butterflies and the word *love* could be found hidden in the castle walls on top of a large butterfly inscribed *LouStrong* underneath. Dan in the Sand is quite famous on the emerald coast for his impressive creations. Onlookers began filling their chairs in a circle, surrounding his work, watching in awe. He explained to wanderers what this sand sculpture represented, resulting in well wishes for me with an occasional similar cancer story. Over the next couple of days, I was able to admire this statue from our balcony, towering in front of the teal blue crystal waters.

Vacation rental prices had skyrocketed since the pandemic had begun. We knew we would not be able to afford to visit the area as often as we were accustomed to prior to my cancer diagnosis. After serious discussion, we made the scary decision to purchase a condo of our own. The remainder of our spring trip was spent driving around in pursuit of the perfect location for us, with the occasional tour. We kept going back to a small complex known as Hermitage by the Bay. It was located on

Okaloosa Island in Fort Walton Beach, Florida, just across the bridge from Destin, in an area that tended to be a little less busy. The location was ideal, across the street from the gulf beaches, sitting on the bay close to Crab Island and included a boat dock. Our dream is to one day own a boat of our own, but in the meantime, we could still rent a vessel for the week. We attempted to put in two offers there, however, lost to a sale before we could even sign the paperwork. With only forty-two units and a tight knit community, it was evident that buying here would be difficult. We continued to look for other options over the next couple of months but our hearts were drawn to that one place. Over the summer, I obtained all of the current owner information from the online tax office. I proceeded to send a letter to every resident that included a short biography of our family as well as our desire to purchase if the time ever would arise that they were interested in selling. Shortly thereafter, we received two messages from owners who were considering selling their properties.

Immediately after arriving to Destin in September, we made a quick stop to feed my mother to calm her hangry, and then we arrived at the Hermitage. This trip included Jean and Al, as well as Megan and her teenage son, Sam. I considered him my bonus son and he often referred to me as *Dad*. Sam enjoyed working out, had curly dark hair and glasses, and to date had never once removed his LouStrong rubber bracelet. We were taken aback as we walked through the first floor door to our prospective new home. Stuck in the eighties, resembling the Golden Girls décor, the walls were covered in a bright pastel peach and the kitchen cabinets painted turquoise. The sectional was geometric shapes of salmon, mint and a dingy ivory, a tall plaster vase lamp covered in dolphins sat on each side. As audacious as it looked, we knew it was merely cosmetic. I could instantly see the potential. We signed the Purchase Agreement that day.

We spent a relaxing week on the water, enjoyed amazing seafood and played card games in the evening that caused us to laugh so hard we often cried. As we spent our final day that week traveling around on the pontoon, taking in one last view of the gorgeous emerald waters, my phone rang. Shawn slowly turned the music off as he watched the joy in my face quickly fade. I had my labs drawn the day before our flight left, however, some of the cancer markers take about a week to result. Dr. Cawley was aware I was on vacation so I knew something was wrong when her voice was on the other end. She let me know that the regimen I had been on the last few months had not been strong enough to keep my kappa numbers down, therefore, I would need to restart the higher dosage again. Definitely not the news I wanted to hear. I begged her to let me attempt to just go back to taking it every day instead of the one week off I had been trying over the last three months. She agreed. After a brief cry, Shawn and I made the decision to put it in the back of our minds, refusing to allow it to ruin our last day. Cranking up the speakers, Shawn pushed the gear to full speed, taking off cruising the bay, my hair blowing in the wind. Our day would come to an end as I was mesmerized by a pod of dolphins surrounding our boat, occasionally jumping out of the water to show off their skills. Being my utmost favorite thing to do here, I could spend hours just watching them swim around us.

One month later, given a week off my chemo, we set off on yet another trip to Florida. This time, however, we would be staying in our new second home. The plan was for Shawn to drive the thirteen hours down in his brown crew cab truck trimmed in camo that was packed full of tools and décor I had purchased in Ohio. Jean and I would fly down to meet him as it was difficult for me to travel long distances. We would only have five full days to renovate an entire two bedroom condo ourselves, as well as hire a contractor to update the bathrooms. I had spent the last couple of weeks strategically ordering furnishings and necessities to arrive over the first few days. Shawn set to work laying new flooring along with most of the other manual labor. My mother began painting the walls and cabinets as well as deep cleaning anything she could get her hands on. I attempted to do as many smaller projects as I was able to do in my condition. I have always loved home projects and was starting to see my vision come together. At one point, Shawn cut off the tip of his finger with a saw. Blood was dripping everywhere. Stubborn and insistent we had no time to waste, he superglued what was left of it back together and went on working. Surprisingly, the chameleon that he apparently is, would regrow that fingertip within weeks. We worked sun up to sun down, only stopping for a quick bite of food we had delivered. This trip would not include sitting by the beach, nor relaxing on a pontoon, but it gave us something more, a home of our own.

By some miracle, we had accomplished a nearly full renovation in less than a week. Walking in, past a wooden mahi fish hanging by the door, our eyes were immediately drawn straight back to the sliding doors overlooking the pool, the dock and the shallow bay water surrounded by mature palm trees towering over the property. The open concept living room and kitchen area was now painted a soft grey to coordinate with the grey wood vinyl plank floors. The kitchen cabinets were now bright white to contrast with the open wood oak shelving displaying teal and white dishes. An ivory island with a wooden walnut top that my dad, a woodworker by trade, had built specifically for our kitchen, sat in the middle next to two amazingly comfortable grey swivel chairs filled with tiny blue specks. I fell in love with these chairs as well as the ability to turn them to face the kitchen or the living room. A canvas of a serene ocean with a faint sailboat in the distance hung above a light blue sofa that held a gel mattress nestled in between two cream end tables topped with gorgeous turquoise blown glass lamps. A long, narrow seafoam console table sat on the side below a navy and grey driftwood whale with coordinating fish. The master bedroom was painted the same color as our bedroom at home, a relaxing light blue called Sparkling Lake. It offered a comfortable king-sized bed with a tufted charcoal headboard and deep teal buttoned bench at the bottom. Two pieces of carved wooden artwork hung in the room, one a happy dolphin, the other a large fish, crafted by a local artisan. A white wooden barn door covered the ensuite bathroom that boasted a newly tiled shower of white, grey and navy, decorated in sea turtle motif. The second bedroom held a full-size bed as well as a low profile twin bunk, covered in white linens, draped with a fun sea creature quilt in coastal colors. The walls were filled with teal and green fish décor. The adjoining bathroom was smaller, with a corner shower, navy blue vanity, decorated with crab artwork. To make it feel more personal for our guests, I made sure to offer children's books about Florida and sea life, board games, beach gear and a fully stocked kitchen. The balcony offered endless views of the vast bay just a short ride away from Crab Island. We named our new home *Mahi Bay* and it was all ours.

The initial plan was for me to ride back with Shawn, stopping for an overnight in Nashville, Tennessee. It just so happened we would be coming through on the fiftieth anniversary of the Grand Old Opry where the show would include several of our favorite artists. Unfortunately, my body gave up all hope of that travel adventure, leaving Jean and I to fly home instead, though this time, treating ourselves to first class for our very worn out bodies. Shawn had known from the beginning there was no way I would make it home with him, but knowing it was on my bucket list, allowed me to maintain hope for that adventure. I will make it there one day.

Shawn and I would make another trip back down in early December to approve the bathroom renovations and finalize any detail before listing our unit on Airbnb. This time, however, I would still be on my daily chemo pill, landing me in bed often during our short stay, struggling with fatigue. I enjoyed the peace and relaxation of this winter trip. We stood in front of Santa's sleigh pulling dolphins on the beach, wearing my blue sweatshirt that read *Who needs Snowflakes when you have Seashells* and a white pair of capris, taking a photo that would become our Christmas card that year. We visited the enormous Christmas tree, surely at least forty feet tall, at Destin

Commons, decorated in red bulbs and red and white striped bows.

Buying a vacation home was a scary venture as we had no idea how well it would do in the rental market. We could not afford to sustain the bills on our own. Much to our surprise, the day our listing went live, bookings began filling the calendar. Thankfully, we would soon find out that it would be easy to maintain bookings throughout the year as well as offer us a free place to stay.

Though still dealing with cancer, as well as the lingering pandemic, this year taught me to accept all of the good with the bad. Wearing masks was still a requirement. Birthdays and holidays were celebrated differently. Graduations were cancelled. The ever-growing list of side effects from having cancer, daily chemo and residual transplant effects would continue. But we made the celebrations work together as a family. We now own a vacation home, something I never thought I would be able to say. I am now an active part of a greater community that thrives for cancer patients. I have been forced to slow down and accept what I cannot change, leaving me incredibly grateful for the days that bring me so much joy.

28

Love & Loss

Christmas was a little different this year because Caleb and his girlfriend both contracted Covid. I tried my best to make spending their first holiday without family nearby a little more comfortable. Still quarantining but feeling better, I ordered a vegan feast and had it delivered for their dinner. We Facetimed to watch them open their stockings that I had sent in the mail. The following week they made the trip down to finish celebrating.

My kappa has continually been increasing, rather than decreasing, with the new dosage, so that has been weighing heavily on our minds. We received the news on Christmas Eve that they were the highest they had been since before transplant. It was devastating news. It was now imperative I resume the higher dosage every single day. Having to learn to deal with the stronger side effects again was beginning to take its toll on me, both physically and emotionally. I am constantly fatigued, exhausted and the simplest things wear me out. Some days, I feel like a boulder is pushing down on my body, deemed as my 'jello days'. I suffer from either insomnia or sleeping most of the day, never getting a regular night's sleep. It was frustrating to feel this incompetent. Chemo brain is for real, causing memory loss and the inability to focus. Every Friday, Shawn fills my plastic rainbow colored weekly pill holders to the brim, twenty-two pills and vitamins every day, not including pain relievers, nausea reducers or muscle relaxers. It quickly became evident my brain was not capable of remembering to take my pills at the specified times. We trained my four-legged genius to not only alert me when it is time to take my pills, but also to retrieve the container for me. I honestly don't know how I would survive without the companionship Joey brings to my life. I was reluctantly learning to adjust to my new chemo regimen.

I had first been introduced to my friend Judy shortly after I was diagnosed. It was surely fate, since a family member told me we should meet AND my social worker suggested Judy be my mentor. Judy is always perfectly tan, petite with short brown hair, thin glasses and the most amazing smile. She had the same type of Multiple Myeloma that I did, but was a little over a year ahead of me in her treatment. The first time I met her was in the parking lot of Walmart, where she fainted right in front of me. She kept apologizing, worried she had frightened me in my early diagnosis. The doctors had still been trying to find the right fit for her medications, which obviously still needed adjusted. Judy was also a breast cancer survivor from years ago but had maintained an inspiring amount of positivity. We quickly developed a close friendship, bonding over a myriad of things only other people going through the same could understand. She lived part of the year here near me in Ohio and the remainder in Florida. Her husband was much like mine, researching cancer updates regularly and treating her like a queen. Judy and I kept in touch weekly, got together for coffee dates and attended Relay for Life with one another. She lives her life to the fullest, succumbing to her bad days, when necessary, all while remaining strong with faith and determination. I admire her strength, her positive attitude and her ability to brighten someone's day with just a smile or a quick note.

Last year, I was introduced by another family member to Kristy, a woman similar in age, who also had Multiple Myeloma. Coincidentally, she was only two weeks ahead of me in her treatment, checking out of transplant just as I was checking in. Kristy was tall with grey hair full of tight curls that she had embraced as it grew back in from her once blonde locks, and was sassy with a great sense of humor. She had two older daughters as well as a younger daughter, all of whom she adored wholeheartedly. It wasn't long before the three of us developed a group chat that offered love, support and a bond unlike any other. The three of us were on the same journey together. Unlike Judy and me, Kristy was diagnosed with lambda, rather than kappa, which was a far more aggressive strand. She knew from the start her battle would be more difficult. And it was. As the year went by, Kristy was increasingly spending more time in the hospital in Columbus. Her immunity numbers kept plummeting, her cancer numbers out of control. She had decided early on that she would take every opportunity to spend her remaining time making memories with her family, especially her younger daughter, which would include trips to Disney and the beach. Kristy had been at the James for a few weeks the beginning of January, trying new chemo regimens and trials. She had finally achieved the numbers she needed in order to participate in one of the newer procedures known as Car-T therapy. Similar to a transplant, yet less invasive, there was hope that eventually this could develop into a cure one day. The following day, her husband called me, his voice shaky. A mold spore had taken over her internally, something her body was too weak to fight off. Her family was saying their final goodbyes. She had come so far to finally get to the point where she was able to harvest cells for the Car-T, only to have something as simple as a mold spore take her life.

I sat on the other end of the phone in shock, trying to find the words to comfort her devastated husband. I am not sure why I was one of the first to be contacted. Perhaps he felt a connection knowing I would understand more than others. Maybe it was because Judy and I had been messaging her often, worried we hadn't heard from her. Whatever the reason, my heart broke for him, for their girls, for the young daughter who would struggle the most. Kristy had fought a hard battle for the last three years, one she ultimately lost. In true fashion, she did not want a funeral, but rather a celebration of life later that summer. I would continue to keep in touch with her family as we were now forever connected by this cancer.

Kristy, Judy and I were all patients of Dr. Bumma. Fully aware of our friendship, he dubbed us "The Triplets". We had now lost one of our trio. Not only did we lose a friend, but that loss also stirred up something else within Judy and I. Our own mortality. We knew Kristy had a more aggressive strand than we had, but in the end, her demise was from a poor immune system that could not fight off something so minuscule that normal people wouldn't even think twice about it. We live with being immunocompromised daily due to the constant chemo. Both Judy and I tend to go down a rabbit hole with our thoughts on occasion and have been known to talk each other down in the late hours of the night when insomnia hits. It was hard to relay to my friends and family my feelings that this could be me in a blink of an eye. The phone call I received from a grieving husband could one day be the call my own husband has to make. Kristy was only diagnosed two weeks before me. I cried through my next appointment with Marcia, who spoke to me a lot about survivor's guilt. My mind was overflowing with so many emotions that I hadn't realized that guilt was one of them. There isn't a week that goes by that I don't think of my friend, her laughter, her family. There are still moments when I pull up our group chat to send a message, forgetting she isn't there to reply.

A couple of weeks later, the nursing home where my grandmother resided notified us that she had contracted Covid and was fading fast. Just minutes after that call, we received news that she had passed away. At ninety-three years old, my Mammy was finally reunited with the love of her life. As heartbroken as I was, I had peace knowing she was where she had wanted to be for the last seven years. She was no longer plagued by the uncertainties of living with dementia. She was laid to rest on Valentine's Day next to my Pappy. I don't think one ever gets over losing a grandparent. There lies a special bond with a grandchild, incomparable to any other. A sage green wooden frame holds a photo of me taken at my wedding, alongside my grandparents I have lost, Bubba, Pappy and Mammy. I look at it every day, a tug at my heart plagued with both love and pain, thankful for the time and memories I was blessed to have with all of them. Another wind chime was added to my front porch, joining the others that represented my guardian angels.

As we said goodbye to my Mammy, we welcomed my niece into this world. Emiliana Sofia was born with a full head of dark hair, just like her brother, and the most adorable chubby cheeks. I was deemed Auntie Annie yet again and I relished the title. Her birth was a much-needed uplifting in a year that had started out full of loss.

Fun fact. Chemotherapy destroys teeth. I loathe anything involving the dentist. Don't get me wrong, I have a great dentist and oral hygienist, but I can't stand anything being done to my teeth. In the first year after diagnosis, I would need eight cavities filled. To make this year even worse to date, pieces of my wisdom teeth began falling out. I had always been told there were nerves wrapped around them so they would be risky to remove. My top two wisdom teeth had grown through properly, whereas my bottom two were impacted, only showing a small amount of enamel through my gums. It was now determined it would be necessary to take that risk. The problem with that was the bone strengthener I had been on for two years prior could cause jaw necrosis from tooth extractions, a very serious and painful jaw bone disfiguration. It had been exactly one year since my last dose but I was still terrified of that possibility. I felt slightly more at ease after I met with an oral surgeon who had been highly recommended to me. It just so happened that Al would also need his wisdom teeth removed the same week as I did. He chose to be brave, staying awake for the procedure, whereas I quickly opted for the twilight option.

The extraction went smoothly. I spent the remainder of the day in bed with Shawn diligently switching out my ice packs from time to time. That night I alternated sweating and freezing while feeling incredibly nauseous. The medications I usually relied on to provide relief of that feeling were not working. My doctor called me in a stronger drug she had just recently began using. My brother and I are both resistant to any medication that is known to cause drowsiness, though often we both wish we could take a pill that would put us out for a good nights' sleep. Much to my surprise, this new drug knocked me out and I was all for sleeping away anything uncomfortable. Unfortunately, it became clear I was suffering from dehydration sickness, unable to keep up with the required sixty-four ounces of daily water intake to combat the chemo. I ended up spending an afternoon at the cancer center receiving an infusion of fluids into my arm. Today, however, would be the first day I would show up empty handed, without baked goods.

My doctors and nurses are constantly working hard to make life easier for every patient. They are required to serve us with long hours with little time off to enjoy themselves. Early on, I began bringing in a variety of trays of sweets as a small token of my appreciation for all they do for us on a daily basis. One of my most enjoyable pastimes has always been cooking and baking. It had become expected of me to shower them with treats at every appointment, their favorite being my famous thumbprint cookies, and I was happy to oblige. After all, they deserved to be spoiled as often as possible. During the weeks I was unable to muster the strength to bake for them myself, I would enlist the help of my mother. When I step off the elevator, the girls at the front desk always exclaim "we saw the baker was coming on the schedule this morning and have been waiting to see what you brought today". It felt good to have another purpose.

29

Enjoying Life Again

A few months ago, a friend of mine sent me a video for the song, "I Believe in You", by JJ Hellar, citing it reminded her of Shawn and me. It followed the daily life of a woman dealing with a serious illness whose husband took care of her and wrote her small notes of encouragement each morning. We have a felt message board in our bedroom with small removable plastic letters that we each take turns leaving notes for one another on. Right now, it reads "You are amazing", a sentiment from my husband. I think it is also imperative that I leave an equal amount of love notes for him so I change it to say "I love your man stank", something I know he will find both funny and endearing. I waited to watch the video until he got home that evening. Immediately, tears began streaming down both our faces as we watched the story unfold, absorbing the words while relating them to our situation, taking them all to heart:

This is not what you thought it would be
Your dreams collide with reality
You're lost in the fog, no answer in sight
You can't find a pill to make it alright
What would I give to make it alright
Running a race with no finish line
Now you're in the fight of your whole life
You work twice as hard to get half as far
I want you to know the hero you are

If you ever start doubting
When it's hard to keep hoping
When you're tired of fighting
And it feels like you're broken
I just want you to know that
I believe in you.

I had never really thought about getting a tattoo before, but as I continued to listen to this song over and over again, an idea came to mind. As another burgundy hair transplant re-birthday was approaching, I made the decision to get my first tattoo. The inside of my left forearm now reads *I Believe in You* in my husband's handwriting overtop a burgundy cancer ribbon fading in to a large butterfly representing my transplant, along with the date of my re-birthday, and three smaller butterflies, each representing another year I have made it through. From this point forward, I plan to add another butterfly to my arm every year on April 17th, my doctors confident I will eventually run out of room. At the same time, Shawn was getting his first tattoo on his upper arm, a black and white tattered flag with a single green stripe representing the military flying above the blue Air Force symbol. Shawn's favorite job of all time was when he was an Air Traffic Controller in England. He had also designed another tattoo on his own, a burgundy cancer ribbon, my transplant date tucked inside the top, fading in to the words *my wife, my life,* completed with a small butterfly. He had this tattoo placed on his heart, right where I will always reside.

This spring, I had been asked to be a model for the Cancer Center fashion show, which raised money for patients who could not afford care, as well as the ability to offer free wigs. Although those closest to me would not consider me shy, I get extremely nervous in front of large crowds. Nevertheless, I was excited for the challenge. My mom and I made a girls' night of it at a small local clothing shop in our historic downtown lined with red brick streets. The owner chose one outfit after another for me to try on, complete with all the coordinating accessories. We had a fun time playing dress up together and Jean insisted on purchasing several items for me to take home after the show.

Each clothing store was granted four models who would be paired together to walk down the runway. Along with myself, our group would include three other amazing women. Dina, a retired teacher with short curly brown hair, thin glasses and the cutest smile, was a long-time cancer survivor. Jeri, who stood tall with long straight blonde hair that had been curled for the occasion, is a newly diagnosed colon cancer patient with the most beautiful soul. Micalyn has shoulder length blonde hair with cat eye glasses and an amazing sense of humor. She had lymphoma several years ago and was currently finishing treatment for tongue cancer. I was fascinated as she showed me the scars on her inner arm where tissue was removed to reconstruct her tongue.

Micalyn, Jeri and I clicked immediately, just as if we had known each other for years, becoming known as the "Blonde Trio". The night of the fashion show, we were all growing increasingly more nervous. Typically, alcohol no longer agrees with my chemo nor my GI tract. Tonight, however, would have to be an exception in an attempt to give me much needed courage. Shawn kept laughing at me as he witnessed my arm moving in and out of the bright red curtain, obtaining glass after glass of Moscato, eventually stealing the whole bottle to sneak to the back to share. Our group was supposed to be at the end of the evening, but the first group had stage fright, which landed us at the front of the line. As music began blowing through the speakers, Micalyn started us all off by heading down the long runway lined with strips of twinkling white lights. I followed behind her lead to the song, "Girl on Fire", by Alicia Keys, My hair was done in several braids overtop my thick blonde curls. Trying not to let my nerves get the best of me, I glanced at Shawn, Jean and Megan who were sitting at a round red table alongside the stage. They were cheering and clapping with smiles wide across their faces as I strolled by. I stepped off the stage only to be greeted by several other friends who were there to support the event. When it was time for my second appearance, I felt a little less scared. I came out to "The Champion", by Carrie Underwood and Ludacris with my hands up in the air, wearing a blue and white striped tank, navy shorts, white sweater cardigan trimmed in red and sapphire stripes, bright white tennis shoes and a large red leather purse. As I began to make the first left turn, I noticed my husband standing at the end of the stage in his grey sweater and light blue cotton pants, waiting for me, his hands tucked in his front pockets. I bent down, softly wrapped my small hands around his face to give him a kiss just as the announcer introduced him to the crowd. All eyes were on us, typically something that would make me incredibly uncomfortable, but in this moment, it was just the two of us. The whole evening was nothing short of amazing. It was becoming clear to me that having cancer would now be an important part of my life, not just all of the negative, but the entire community that embodies our group as a whole. I was celebrated tonight by an entire auditorium full of other women filling the room with nothing but pure encouragement. It was an amazing feeling. To top it off, I was also leaving with several new friends, certain that we would remain in each other's lives.

My entourage, consisting of Shawn, Megan and Jean, along with a couple of her girlfriends, cried the majority of the show. Tears of both happiness and sadness listening to all of the survivors' stories filled them with emotions. Some had been in remission for years, while others were terminal, living out their final days. My mom would later tell me it was evident that Shawn was overjoyed watching me strut down the runway while smiling, laughing with my new friends and sneaking wine. Some husbands would be bored in this scenario or even jealous that my time wasn't being spent with him. Not mine. He was genuinely happy that I was enjoying a night of normality. Inspired by the amazing women I had befriended that evening, I returned home with new confidence that I had been lacking over the last several months.

Still off chemo allowing my mouth to recover from my wisdom teeth removal, I decided to take full advantage of feeling better. We spent a long weekend in Pigeon Forge, Tennessee, relaxing in a cabin, fulfilled with each other's company. We enjoyed the mountains, good food and a quiet ride on the lake. A few weeks after, we were able to meet up with Shawn's parents at our condo in Florida. It was a perfect week. May is my favorite time of the year to visit. The weather was amazing, the water crystal clear teal the entire time. The dolphins were plentiful, constantly swimming around our pontoon with the occasional baby calf alongside its mother. I could sit and watch them all day long and be perfectly content. We had become very comfortable in our new second home, not wanting to leave.

As summer began and my chemo break was coming to an end, we scheduled a trip to Columbus for the weekend. We spent the day watching the Memorial Golf Tournament, keeping an eye out for my favorite golfers. Still difficult for me to walk long distances, we chose a spot directly inside the gates to sit our chairs for this beautiful sunny day. The last time we had been to a golf match was only a few months prior to my diagnosis. I was happy to be able to attend a course again.

The next morning, we headed to a park downtown near the James hospital to attend my first in person Muscles for Myeloma walk. When we arrived, we were overwhelmed by the parking lot full of other Multiple Myeloma patients and their supporters all wearing the same hunter green shirts that read *Moves for Myeloma* in white. Our cancer ribbon color is burgundy so I have never figured out why these shirts are always green, but nevertheless, we were all advocating together. Several people were cheering us on through megaphones, handing out a variety of fun things to add to our gift bags and encouraging us to take photos. I held a large poster frame in front of me that had been decorated for the event as well as a cardboard bubble that read *Survivor* for my photo op. As the bullhorn sounded, my hand gripped firmly in my husband's, we took off slowly to complete our lap. The path was gorgeous, fully engulfed in tall trees full of lush leaves that hovered together over top of us. A few minutes later, we would cross the finish line under an inflatable green arch covered in butterflies. My body ached but my heart was full. Dr. Bumma was waiting at the end to congratulate his patients as they completed their lap one by one. Today, I was surrounded by nothing but support and encouragement by people dealing with the same cancer. Some part of me needed this feeling. We spent the rest of the morning exchanging stories with other survivors, once again taking in this new community I was embracing this year.

Shortly after I resumed the Revlimid, we took a short trip to visit Bruce and Carol in Myrtle Beach, South Carolina. It was peaceful and relaxing just to spend time with them. On our final day, we drove down to Charleston where we toured the town in a horse drawn carriage and explored the market. Later that year, for Christmas, my mother-in-law bought me a gorgeous straw basket handmade by the women in that market that carried an aroma of fresh hay. The heat, as well as the exertion on my body, wore me down, quickly forcing us to head back early. Shawn kept reminding me that I needed to accept the good days with the bad. After all, I had been blessed with several good days over the last two months.

I had packed as many excursions in as I could over the last few weeks off chemo. I may not have been able to eat normally quite yet but I was determined not to let that stop me from taking full advantage of my time off. Originally, it was thought I would need to add the Velcade belly shots back for a bit to get things under control, however, due to an unforeseen infusion of Dex during my surgery, it helped to keep my numbers controlled for a brief time. I was grateful for the trips we were able to take, the new friends I had made and the cancer community I was increasingly immersing myself in.

30

Defeated

It was evident that my body was not accepting of the poison that I was once again forcing inside me. I was unable to get out of bed for days. My body felt like jello, like a weight was sitting on top of me that I couldn't get out from under. I was becoming overly frustrated. The last few weeks I was reminded of what it felt like to be off chemo. Now, I was feeling worse than ever. Everything hurt. My right hand had become so shaky that I was dropping anything I attempted to hold. I was tired. So incredibly fatigued. My brother once told me when you are feeling terrible it makes everything else seem much worse, even the smallest things. I had been given a reminder of how my former life used to feel, only to have it taken away. I was struggling with that acceptance while my body was rejecting the toxins.

My doctors here scheduled several tests in an attempt to find the cause of my hand tremors. My kappas were continuing to rise. Reluctantly, I tried medical marijuana gummies for the pain. Although they provided some relief, I hated the way they made me feel. I was already fatigued all of the time and I felt like the drug just made that worse. My husband, the world's best caregiver, was forced to sit beside the bed, day after day, watching his wife slip away to darkness. My face had grown even more ghostly, the shadows expanding underneath my eyes, my body becoming more frail as I began withering away to nothing, unable to maintain an appetite. There were days I would catch him crying when it became unbearable for him to watch me suffer. Knowing how miserable I was and being unable to fix it for me was killing him inside. One night we were watching a music award show on TV and Taylor Swift began singing acapella with a piano. As the lyrics continued on, tears ran down his face.

> *You make the best of a bad deal*
> *I just pretend it isn't real*
> *Soon you'll get better*
> *'cause you have to*
> *What am I supposed to do*
> *If I don't have you*

My husband will tell you that I am the strongest person in the world, but that night, as I watched him crumble inside, it was him who was the strongest through his weakness. It was he who had to stand by with a broken heart, day after day, using his strength as my rock. His suffering was my fault.

My MRI was done at Ohio State two days before my previously scheduled appointment. It happened to be our wedding anniversary so we decided to make the best of it by booking a hotel in Dublin, close to Columbus, for a couple of nights while we were there. I began the first day dressed in a ridiculously oversized gown and pants that could have fit four of me in them to get my imaging. Afterwards, we celebrated our wedding date with a romantic dinner at a restaurant called *The Barn*. We enjoyed lobster bisque and the most amazing smoked pork chop, still on the bone, that somehow tasted like charred pork, ham and bacon together as one. The meal was nothing short of amazing. Following our dinner, we visited my brother and his family so we could enjoy a little time with our niece and nephew. I was beyond exhausted but I have always told myself I would push as far as humanly possible, knowing the outcome would be miserable, to enjoy time with those two babies. They make my heart so incredibly happy.

Everything caught up with me the next morning and I knew most of my day would be spent in bed. We went out for coffee, explored the historic downtown a bit and found two amazing waterfalls right off the road. I could have stayed to admire the rush of water forcing down over the slick rocks spraying me with cool mist for hours but my body was telling me otherwise. The remainder of the day would be spent in bed at the hotel. We ordered pizza rather than going out for dinner that evening to have a quiet night in. I fell asleep early, allowing me to succeed in a good night's rest.

The next day, I had an appointment with Dr. Bumma where I explained to him all of the difficulties I was having since resuming the Revlimid. He questioned me "What is the point of fighting and taking chemo if you never have a good quality of life?" These are words that I will never forget. Though it was evident a lower dose was not enough to control my cancer, he was willing to let me try to take the pill for three weeks followed by one week off every month to allow my body to recover from the havoc wreaking inside me from the chemo. I was excited for this change although scared of the possibility it would not be enough as my kappa continued to rise. I was so miserable that I was willing to try anything. My off week would not be for a couple more weeks so that it would coincide with the new tattoo I had scheduled.

The day after we returned from our trip to Columbus, I was home alone while Shawn was at work. A severe pain tore across my chest bringing me quickly down to my knees on the floor. Not wanting to alarm anyone, I laid on the floor, Joey's warm body pressed against me, for several minutes waiting for the pain to subside. When it was clear it was not going to ease, I called my brother who did not answer. I finally gave in to phone my mother who flew down the driveway in a cloud of dust. In the meantime, Chad had called me back, explaining to me it was most likely due to the cervical issues that had also been causing my hand tremors. I sat on my knees, bent over, tears pouring down my face and desperately whispering to my brother that I did not want to do this anymore. Silence was on the other end, followed by "I know", unsure of how to comfort me at that time, knowing there was nothing he could say to make it better. Jean ran through the house to my bedroom to find my head over the toilet. The pain was so severe that it was making me sick. My brother advised her of what medication to find in my small personal pharmacy to administer to me when I was able to keep them down. After two more trips to the bathroom, my mother helped me to bed, gave me my pills, laid the heating pad on my neck and tucked me in under the warmth of my electric blanket. Just like my Bubba used to do to her, she filled a bowl with cold water floating with ice cubes. Unable to hold back her emotions, my mother cried as she tediously moved the washcloth back and forth between my forehead and the bowl. This was never going to end. There would always be a reason for her daughter to need a caregiver. I begged them both not to call Shawn as I knew he was on an important conference call at a store several miles away. Neither of them listened to me so I received a frantic call from him as soon as he got the messages. He was devastated that he was not here to take care of me. By the time he arrived home, things had settled down and my medicines had kicked in.

The last several weeks had left me feeling defeated. I did not want to do the things that don't kill me but make me stronger anymore. I was ready to give up and throw in the towel. Shawn encouraged me to just ignore the doctors and take a chemo break now. It wasn't worth how miserable it was making me. In true form, I told him I was fine. I was determined to make it to my newly scheduled off week.

They say after you get your first tattoo you become addicted. When Megan asked me to get a matching one with her, I was on board right away. We decided on a small bouquet of flowers on our inner right arms that included both our birth month flowers. Mine was April, which were sweet pea and daisy. Hers, being November, were chrysanthemum and peony. It was clear as soon as the artist began that this time around wouldn't be as successful. I was bleeding everywhere, leaving a large, swollen puddle of blood underneath my skin. Apparently, being off chemo for only a couple of days is not long enough to get a tattoo. It took me a few days to recover from that ordeal, but afterward I was able to admire my new floral tattoo with just the tiniest amount of color shaded inside.

Over the next couple of weeks, I consulted with several neurosurgeons regarding my neck. I had known early on that another back surgery would be necessary, putting it off, blaming Covid. The neck situation, however, was a new occurrence. It was now becoming obvious that I would require a cervical surgery as well. To be honest, I was terrified to do either one. Some of the surgeons were less comfortable than others, citing the uncertainty if the fusion would hold due to the lesions on my spine, both now and in the future in the case that new ones would arise. We had a lot of decisions to make. In the meantime, I would continue to receive steroid shots in my hips and shoulders in order to mask some of my joint pain. I had always heard horror stories about the long needles inserted deep inside, however, they did not seem terrible to me. Maybe I was just used to pain, though unsure if I will ever be used to the needles, or I just have a great orthopedic doctor, who also is a longtime friend. I had been advised to drink pickle juice to combat muscle aches as well as assist with hydration, something that, despite my best efforts, I often was lacking. I have always loved pickles of all kinds. I remember when I was a young girl crawling into my Bubba's bed, curling up with her and a bowl of dill spears watching the show, *Dallas*. At this point, I was willing to try just about anything for relief so I began intaking the sour juice daily.

I was over three years out of transplant but most days I still felt terrible. The first thing I feel every morning is the piercing ache from my joints and muscles. My body stays in a state of constant pain of varying degrees. Neuropathy plagues my feet and hands. I seem to suffer from insomnia most nights with the occasional days where I am only awake a few hours. The constant fatigue and exhaustion are often discouraging, being forced to rest while replaying a list of things I wanted to accomplish instead. My nausea, loss of appetite and weight loss is always a cause for concern by my doctors due to my protein intake, or lack thereof. I usually offer up a wrinkle of my nose when I am urged to eat more food and more often. The Revlimid is infamous for its ability to remove everything from my body as soon as I ingest it. On top of the hiatal hernia I have, the chemo has wreaked havoc on my GI system, making it even more difficult to maintain certain foods such as raw fruits and vegetables. I needed the transplant for a deeper response to my cancer with the hope it would be able to be managed longer, however, years later I was still struggling from its side effects together with the daily chemo. Medicine that was supposed to heal me continues to destroy parts of me. At what point does suffering through the plethora of side effects just to stay alive become too much for one to bear without giving up entirely?

I had been losing faith fast over the last two months, but cautiously eager to start my new off week routine, hoping it would bring me some much-needed relief, even if only for a short while.

31
My People

A few months ago, my cancer friends and I began a daily group chat for support, encouragement and in general conversation. It consisted of myself, Judy, Micalyn, Jeri, Missy and April. Missy was diagnosed with neuroendocrine pancreatic cancer two years ago. She was strong and resilient, constantly running her three children around to sports and school events. April was a friend of Jeri's who was currently battling breast cancer. We had decided we would all attend Relay for Life together. Missy, however, was struggling with going, feeling like she was not a survivor, given her cancer was terminal. I urged her to go, citing that she was still here fighting, surviving two years thus far. I have said many times in the past that I was incredibly grateful I was diagnosed after Caleb graduated so that he did not have to watch me struggle daily. I was glad I did not have to sacrifice missing sports games, music or school events and all the little things like driving him and his friends around town. My heart ached for Missy's internal struggle but I admired her perseverance and her determination to spend all the time she was able to making memories with her children. In the end, she decided to attend the event, forming friendships and finding the support she was lacking.

The evening of Relay for Life could not have been more perfect, sunny with a light breeze just as the sun was going down. This would be the first time all six of us would spend time together in person. We wore matching purple shirts that read *Survivor* across the back above the phrase *Celebrate, Remember, Fight Back* in white. I had made decals on my Cricut of each of our colored cancer ribbons to iron on our sleeves, mine and Judy's being burgundy. Although some of us shared the same cancers, we were brought together by a common struggle no matter what the diagnosis. We all belong to an exclusive club, one that none of us signed up for.

After a short introduction speech followed by a group photo of all the patients attending the evening, we gathered together for the survivors walk. The song, "Just Stand Up", an upbeat medley from several female artists recorded for a Stand Up to Cancer event, began blaring through the speakers.

The heart is stronger than you think
It's like it can go through anything
And even when you think it can't
It finds a way to still push on, though
Sometimes you wanna run away
Ain't got the patience for the pain
And if you don't believe it, look into your heart
The beat goes on.
I'm tellin' you, things get better, through whatever
If you fall, dust it off, don't let up
Don't you know you can go be your own miracle
If the mind keeps thinking you've had enough
But the heart keeps telling you don't give up
Who are we to be questioning
Wondering what is what

Don't give up
Through it all, just stand up
You got it in you, find it within you
The order of the line up was organized by the number of years we had survived, most of us fitting in to the less than three year category but all choosing to stay together. We began our short walk around the park, smiling sheepishly at the crowd surrounding us cheering, uncomfortable being the center of attention. White and lavender luminaries filled with bright candles lined the path, each with a name representing either a survivor or in memory of. We sought out to find our names, those we love and those we've lost. Along with mine, I located one for Al, one for Shawn's good friend who was currently in treatment for Hodgkin's Lymphoma, as well as the one I had purchased for my dear friend, Kristy, wishing she was here with us. I embraced familiar faces I had located in the crowd, friends and survivors from my past. My mother cried from the sidelines, eagerly wanting to embrace me but fighting restraint, allowing me to have this moment with my gals.

Dr. Cawley was the guest speaker this year. There wasn't a single dry eye in our group as she preached for a better tomorrow. That woman is nothing short of remarkable. We smiled through several photo sessions holding up glittered signs including one that read "Cawley's Cancer Crew" that we held in front of our beloved doctor. We visited the survivor booth where we filled our bags with a variety of cancer related and encouraging goodies. Every year, we are awarded a gold star pin with the current year stamped across the middle to add to the purple medal hanging around our neck. This would be my fourth star, a reward for making it one more year.

Many attendees spent the remainder of the evening visiting the different booths or bidding on silent auctions. Our group found a remote spot to gather around. For what seemed like hours, we sat uncomfortably on hard metal white chairs, chatting about the things we couldn't with our regular friends. You can't really say "raise your hand if you have pooped your pants from chemo" to 'normal' friends. We could all relate to what one another had been through or was going through now. We shared remedies with each other that we had personally found successful in the hopes it could be helpful to another. I am certain we all felt a sense of relief being able to release all the emotions we had been feeling without the typical "I'm fine" response. As the sun moved to darkness, we continued to laugh and share stories, feeling as if we had all been friends for years. We were diagnosed with different cancers, but we all suffered similar side effects as well as the mental and physical struggles.

When one is first diagnosed, everyone is eager to support you in any way that they can, while offering a constant rush of encouragement. If you are lucky, you go through initial treatment, succeed in a remission with the hope you can put it all in the past, for it never to return again. If you suffer from the worst diagnosis, you are given a timeframe of what you have left on this earth in the best case scenario. If you fall somewhere in the middle, as I do, you live in a constant state of treatment, cancer always looming in the background. You may feel grateful you haven't been given a number, though wishing in the back of your mind you were one of those luckier ones. As time goes by, it becomes awkward for people to have conversations about it, unsure of what exactly to say. "Well, you look good," could possibly be one of the worst compliments to give a cancer patient, though given out of sincerity by loved ones who are unsure of what to say. That may, in fact, be true, however, the majority of the time it is just a brave face to avoid the awkwardness of revealing all the things you don't see. An attendee at Relay offered that phrase to a friend of mine who had lost nearly one hundred pounds due to her illness. She was offended by the compliment of her weight loss due to her condition. It was not meant as such, but to her, it is a constant reminder of how she appears now. It is difficult for family and friends to watch you struggle all of the time, not knowing what to say, resulting in communication often dissipating. It isn't that they don't care, it is just a really difficult thing to watch others suffer.

As the evening came to an end, I looked around our circle, watching my girls smile and laugh, certain it was the most we had all let loose in quite a long time. These women were my people, my tribe, what I needed in my life. I knew from this point on we had found the support we could only achieve from each other. The time had come for the closing survivors' walk. When I stood up, it was immediately clear that my hips and back would fail to cooperate, unable to complete that final path. It was fine though, I did not feel defeated that night. I was uplifted by these people. Shawn put his arm around me to help me to the car, kissed my forehead while exclaiming just how proud he was of me. He had spent the evening with a couple of the other husbands, patiently waiting for us girls to finish our talk. My mom would later gush about how content she was to catch him watching me from across the park, a big smile plastered across his face. My husband's heart melts when he sees me happy. Later on, I would find out from another husband, who had asked him how long we were staying, Shawn's reply was "However long she wants to stay and if she wears herself out too much, I will just carry her to the car".

This year was continuing to show me that no matter how hard of a struggle some days could be, I needed more than my inner circle. My family and friends were amazing, but I was part of something bigger now. Cancer would be a part of me for the remainder of my life here on Earth. I found myself embracing that community more and more this year.

32
Roller Coaster

As I have come to realize, this cancer is much like a roller coaster ride. It often feels like I take two steps forward to be pushed ten steps back. There will always be good days along with the bad. My cancer, at times, will be more stable than others, resulting in a constant realignment in my regimen. I have learned to be more accepting of this realization but often times it is still frustrating. There have been days where I have looked at my husband and uttered the words "I feel so normal today…if only this would last" and others when I was ready to give up. The constant waiting for test results is enough to drive a sane person crazy. Every month, refreshing the app on my phone every fifteen minutes, anxiously waiting to see what this month looks like, is exhausting. My husband once said to me that it was a daily mental tear that never goes away and he was absolutely correct. As summer began to fade away, it was evident that this new season would bring along quite the ride, leaving nothing to be easy.

I grew up with the privilege of spending most of my time surrounded by a remarkable family who loved me dearly. My Aunt Regina, who has gorgeous long white hair, has lived in Colorado for several decades now. I am her only niece, leaving her to dote on me often. My Uncle Bill, tall with thinning dark hair, who now resides a state away, is an Army veteran who affectionately called me

"Bird Legs" when I was a skinny little girl, then somewhere over the years changed it to "Schnook". Uncle Cliff, a former Navy man with his growingly bald head and giant grin, who calls me "Annie", and his wife, Aunt Ann with dark brown hair full of tight curls and a sweet personality, have always had a strong presence in my life. They all hold a heart full of gold that wished nothing but the best for me. I am beyond thankful to have them all in my life. They would provide me with wonderful cousins and, although I love them all, I am especially close to Whitney, who shares her mother's tight curls in lighter brown hair, her father's big smile and hazel green eyes that mimic my own. She is blessed with two beautiful daughters, who I refer to as my nieces, even though that technically isn't the correct title. Ryleigh is the younger of the two, always eager to help. McKenzie is quickly becoming a teenager still holding on to her inner child. They both share perfectly tan skin, long wavy brown hair and baby blue eyes. Although those characteristics alone do not resemble mine, we have always said that somehow McKenzie could pass as my daughter with our similarities. I had been promising my two 'nieces' for weeks they could have a sleepover, but up until now, I had been increasingly miserable. We finally set a date only for one of them to wake up with a stuffy nose the night before. Fully aware and understanding of my situation at such a young age, she instantly burst into tears with the thought of not being able to have our night together. I contacted my doctor who advised me that she most likely had a cold that I would probably get but could fight off. I chose to get sick over breaking these girls' hearts who I love so very much. We spent an entire evening crafting, tie dying shirts, scrapbooking photos from our evening then cuddling up in bed watching movies. Those girls wore me out beyond exhaustion but I loved every minute of it. They would return with their mom a few months later to bake Christmas cookies together from the recipe passed down from Bubba: soft and thick, sour cream sugar cookies with a pinch of nutmeg, decorated to perfection. There was never a year we did not bake hundreds of them with our grandmother and I was not about to lose this tradition.

A couple weeks later, on the evening before our flight down on another September trip to our second home, I noticed some swelling around my eye. Not concerned, but taking the proactive approach, knowing I would be in Florida for the next week, I reached out to my doctor, wondering if it could be a spider bite. I was advised to apply a bit of steroid cream I had on it and to send an updated photo to her in the morning. When I awoke, it had spread, was fiercely red around bubbles that appeared full of fluid. Ugh. Can't things ever be easy anymore? My phone rang immediately after sending the new photo. I had shingles. It was a race between my doctor and my husband in order to get the medicine filled and obtained prior to our departure. Luckily, we had an afternoon flight. It was imperative I start treatment right away to prevent the spread inside my eye. Over the next couple of days, it would extend to the side of my face and slightly back into my hair. Thankfully, we had caught it early, managing to keep it under control. I made a point to stick my head down in the warm salt water every now and then in an attempt to dry up the sores. I hid them behind my white aviator sunglasses with shiny blue polarized lenses. They were extremely painful, however, I tried to focus on enjoying our vacation, this time learning to balance on our new paddle board. We all had a few nosedives in the water. It wasn't nearly as easy as it may seem. Watching Joey enjoy the pontoon rides, his wet fur slicked back by the wind, wearing his blue doggie goggle sunglasses, was enough to make anyone smile. He loved boat rides just as much as we did. On our final day, we got caught up in a downpour just before we made it back to the condo. We were all soaked from head to toe. As we disembarked the boat, with it still being warm outside, I gave in to the rain, splashing barefoot in the deep puddles overflowing the sidewalks, water streaming down over my favorite floral rain jacket in varying shades of teal. In this moment, I was a carefree child again.

I had shingles once before in my mid-twenties. Just prior to that, I was having some abnormal labs, resulting in a leep procedure from my gynecologist. At the time, I had no energy and randomly fell asleep even while sitting up. When I first noticed the red and purple patches on my side, bottom and hip, they appeared as bruises but quickly became bursts of sharp pain shooting down my legs. When it had become unbearable, unfortunately over a weekend, I was forced to be seen at the emergency room. Through my objections, that doctor told me I had carpet burn. I asked him what in the world he thought I was doing at home. Yep, a five-hundred-dollar copay for that diagnosis. I left still in pain and extremely annoyed. The following morning, I went to my primary care physician, who informed me that I had shingles, which was rare for someone of my age. Looking back, we have often wondered if my Smoldering Myeloma or MGUS, the predecessor to full blown Multiple Myeloma, was just beginning.

Continuing on this roller coaster into fall, I was over the moon with excitement we were able to have Applefest this year. This fall celebration on the farm has been in existence well before my mom married into the family and something everyone looked forward to in October every year. It is a day shared with over one hundred family and friends, cooking apple butter in a copper pot over the fire, soup beans in a cast iron kettle, apple cider from an antique press and so much more. Al and Jean had been unable to host this event for the last two years due to the pandemic. The pole barn was filled with smoked meat, endless side dishes warming in crock pots and a wall of tables lined with decadent desserts. Shawn's parents always drive up for the occasion, this year bringing along a gorgeous round cake with an apple tree on it. Applefest was a day to spend with so many of our loved ones all together in one location, which to me, was all that mattered. This year, it would be sunny, sixty-five degrees, leaves boasting gold and orange, the quintessential perfect fall day.

Autumn is my favorite time of the year and I was bound and determined to do all of the things on my bucket list that I missed out on last year. We enjoyed weekend trips along with outdoor food and craft festivals. Our date nights consisted of dinner in the park surrounded by freshly fallen leaves or movie nights with milkshakes in bed. I participated in a Move Mountains 5K walk downtown to benefit cancer research at the James with my Blonde Trio, although Micalyn and I were both having a bit of a down day, therefore not making it far. A local farm offers phenomenal photo backdrops consisting of a floral mum wall, a tower of wood crates filled with pumpkins and gourds, a hay bale transformed in to a giant golden sunflower, along with many others. Being the photography loving gal that I am, navigating all the photo opportunities is something I love to do every year so I was happy to resume that tradition.

Jean was busy putting up wallpaper in my house this month, a gorgeous turquoise grass cloth in my craft room and an amazing baby blue one, boasting with large yellow flowers on my laundry room ceiling, both turning out amazing. In an attempt to assist her by finding something in my toolbox, I managed to fall over a pile on the floor, causing injury to both my neck and back. I was immediately sent for imaging to determine if I had fractured anything again, which thankfully I had not. Normal people would baby the pain for a few days to see if it lessens, but given my condition, it is always imperative that even the smallest of things are checked out right away.

It had been four years since my last concert. We had made the decision to purchase tickets for a Justin Moore concert, one that we had to miss out on shortly after my diagnosis. It was a smaller venue about a little over an hour away. As the time was quickly approaching, we became nervous about my first indoor outing among a crowd. I had not been feeling the best over the last two days, plagued with fatigue, but I was determined to make this concert. We enjoyed a dinner of wood fired pizza then checked into the hotel which was only a couple blocks away from the venue. Running behind, I neglected to take time to rest up a bit before heading over to find our third row aisle seats at center stage. A wave of excitement rushed over my husband and I as we eagerly awaited him to arrive on stage. After all, he was one of our favorite artists, one we had not yet seen in person. Once he appeared, we sang along to every song, knowing all of them by heart, hips swaying from side to side. My husband embraced me and began serenading me when *With a Woman you Love* came on, only to be pulled away by his new bromance from across the aisle, a young muscular guy, clearly drunk. As the night went on, I began feeling worse, suffering from exhaustion and stomach pain, causing me to sit down, the only person in a chair surrounded by a room of concert goers standing up cheering for the country singer on stage. I was embarrassed. I felt as if everyone was staring at me wondering what was wrong with me, well aware it was most likely all in my head. Shawn kept insisting we leave, which I pushed back with "I'm fine", determined I was not going to ruin this night for him. There came a point where he was no longer going to accept my persistence.

My husband would carry me back to the hotel, tears streaming down my face, disappointed with how the evening had panned out. I wanted this night to be as normal as it would have been before I had cancer. I wanted to sing, dance and get lost in the effects of beer. I had ruined our much anticipation return to concert life. Shawn continued to reiterate how much fun we had, insisting I was being ridiculous as he tucked me into bed, offering me my pain meds. In an attempt to make me smile, he will often do a little shuffle across the room or make up a dance routine. There was nothing he could do or say to me to make me think otherwise. Nothing was ever easy anymore.

A couple days later, right before Thanksgiving, we realized we had contracted the flu that was plaguing our town. Shawn began showing signs first so as soon as I began coughing, I contacted my doctor, who immediately sent me for testing. There was currently a trifecta of Covid, Influenza A and RSV strong in adults this year. As soon as it was confirmed that I did indeed have the flu, she put me on medication right away. It was too far out for Shawn to benefit, which led to me recovering before my husband. We were bedridden and miserable for a few days but spent the time binge watching some of our favorite shows which included The Crown. I have always enjoyed historical monarchy movies. Interestingly, the news reported that Queen Elizabeth, who had just recently passed away, was actually suffering from Multiple Myeloma as well over her last year. If that is indeed true, how crazy would that be?

There aren't many tangible things I need in my life as I prefer experiences instead of physical gifts. For Christmas this year, Shawn gifted me an overnight stay at a nearby lodge that included an outdoor dinner in a heated igloo. Overly excited about the adventure, we checked in a couple of days after the holiday. The room was huge, decorated with deer motif and a large sectional sofa in the corner next to the second floor balcony that overlooked the snow covered gardens with the faint sound of waterfalls in the distance. The king size bed now topped my list of the softest, most plush, comfortable bed I have ever laid on, resulting in me attempting to buy one for home, though I was unsuccessful. Our igloo sat in a corner, covered in white lights, filled with a basket of blankets and a Bluetooth speaker so that we may choose our own music. The dinner consisted of creamy butternut squash soup, a cherry salad, smoked stuffed chicken and finished with a warm apple dumpling and a hot chocolate bomb slowly melting in a mug. Throughout the night I had pain in my neck that was progressively becoming worse as I attempted to keep it to myself, determined to have a romantic evening with my amazing husband. Unsuccessful in that attempt, Shawn suggested we make an early night of it, ran me a hot bubble bath and retrieved my pain pills. I was so looking forward to a wonderful night's sleep in that dreamy bed that I fell fast asleep. I awoke in the middle of the night screeching in severe pain radiating from my neck up through the back of my head. I took another pain pill with no relief. I have become ridiculously pain tolerant but this particular ache was something I had been unable to control. As the sun was beginning to rise, we made the decision to head home. Shawn helped me to the car, handed me a coffee and covered me in the heated blanket I keep in the car. Tears flowed down my face, both from the pain, as well as the shame. Once again, I had ruined another evening for my husband. He wiped my face, stared me dead in the eyes, insisting we had an amazing evening together, that I was being too hard on myself. By the time we reached Marietta, my doctor had ordered an emergency MRI and suggested I begin alternating different pain meds to find relief. Over the years, I have become quite good at suffering through pain, often times without anyone noticing. This pain was reminiscent of my initial diagnosis. In the end, it was determined that picking up my nephew, who was over three times my weight limit allowance, as well as crawling back and forth in a toddler's play tunnel, had irritated my already bulging discs in my neck just enough to cause such piercing pain. I adore my niece and nephew and would do anything in the world for them, therefore, I often ignore my restrictions when it comes to playing with them. I have always had the mindset that the temporary additional discomfort that may come with me overdoing it is far worth it in the end. Spending time being an Auntie is more important. However, it was now becoming evident that I could no longer avoid my impending neck surgery.

As the year drew to a close, I felt more defeated than I had in a long time. It seemed like everything I tried to do that resembled a pre-cancer normal was inevitably ruined by something new due to my current condition. There comes a point where you no longer care if there is a light at the end of the tunnel or not. You're just sick of the tunnel. Shawn was constantly reminding me of all the things we did this year as well as the trips we took that were successful, although most of those were while I was off the chemo for several weeks. Maybe that was the problem. I had a taste of my old life, the one before cancer. Perhaps I craved what I had before, knowing I would never go back to that life. My life was not supposed to turn out this way. My husband was right though. This was the first year since diagnosis followed by the pandemic that I was able to return to doing things I had previously enjoyed. They may not have all turned out to be a complete success, but in the end, it was far better than not being able to do them at all. My final thought of the year would come from Megan, who sent me an emotional text with a resolution to do all of the things we always say we are going to do whenever I am able to do so. I accepted the challenge.

33

What You Don't See

As with other blood cancers, Multiple Myeloma just doesn't go away. There is no cure, only harsh treatments that keep me alive while trying to balance a good quality of life. It is a cancer where no two patients are alike. I was told once by my doctor that one of my friends was doing really well, another doing poorly and I resided somewhere in the middle. I am not complaining. I am lucky to still be on this Earth. My heart aches for those who do not have the options that I do, only to be left counting down their remaining days. I often fantasize what my life would be like if I had a cancer that just went away after a few months of treatments. As the years go by it is far easier to tell people two simple words: "I'm fine", portraying the version of me that I want people to see. The times I do get to travel, to share experiences and all of the things I am able to do. I want others to see me as I used to be, not the me who struggles daily. I am the strong woman, not the one who silently cries in the shower only to step out as super woman. On the other side of that, I think it becomes easy for people to forget I even have cancer, thanks to photo filters masking my chemo eyes, as well as my long blonde hair that thankfully my current regimen does not strip from me. It is easier to remember someone has cancer when they are bald. What I struggle with the most is what you don't see.

Some days are easier than others, but the truth is, usually I am not fine. I am fighting internally to get by the best way I know how. Inside, I often want to crawl under my heated blanket, curl up in anguish, wishing the day away. I don't want anyone to know otherwise, seeing me as weak, when I so badly want to portray myself as strong. Sometimes it is easier to say "I'm fine" rather than spend what little energy I possess now explaining why I am not. There are times my brain is overwhelmed and I am unable to focus my mind, but I try to stay positive so that I don't bring others down with me. Who actually wants to hear over and over again that I feel miserable? And if they do, how does one continue to find the proper words to respond? My family has learned my tells from my chemo eyes and my silence. Never being one to complain about pain until it becomes unbearable, I often stay quiet to work through it.

Imagine living your busy daily life, waking up late for work running out the door, coming home to running your children around to sports and activities, getting dinner together and finishing all the household chores before bed. Life is bustling day after day boasting with human social interactions. You wake up one day only to find out that your body has begun to betray you. All of the daily activities you took for granted now knock all the wind out of you. Suddenly, you are endlessly tired, feeling as if a boulder is forcing down on your entire body, resulting in the need to use up all of your energy just to get out of bed. Guilt quickly takes over as you feel lazy, unable to complete daily tasks. You feel failure as you are no longer able to provide for your family in the capacity you did before, believing you are letting them all down. Your body is weak, so weak that it takes so much strength to accomplish just about anything. Spending a day out shopping could land you in bed for a couple of days to recover. You live in a constant suffering state of pain, not allowed to take normal relief medications for fear of blood clots. There is a constant struggle to take narcotics to mask the pain while feeling guilty for taking them. The stigma around controlled substances is always negative. Addiction is a real and frightening disease. If you give in to taking them, will you become an addict? Four years in, it became obvious for me that I did not carry that gene, however, it is still a constant mental battle whether or not to take them when I am suffering, even though I know they will provide much needed relief.

Your frail bones are now riddled with lesions and easily breakable. The fogginess in your brain makes you lose all focus, leaving you enormously frustrated, unable to convey what you really mean the majority of the time. You constantly apologize to others when you get lost carrying on a conversation. The drugs cause you to fill with a wide array of emotions often closing them in without an outlet. Every waking moment is a battle using your smile as your shield. Life inevitably moves on without you. You hide your struggles in an effort not to burden those closest to you. You crave human interaction full of normal conversation. Between treatment and the pandemic, you live alone in isolation the majority of the time.

People often question how I do it every day. I wasn't given a choice. I did not ask to have cancer. The only option was to fight or give up. It is easier to smile and pretend I am okay than the alternative. I live in a world of survival mode. More than anything, I reside in a state of pure exhaustion, both physically and mentally. I am strong but I am also tired. I am battling things every day that I will never share with you. Sometimes I feel like I have been drained of everything I have to give. That doesn't stop me from fighting nor does it keep me from living. Sometimes I am forced to make concessions all while learning to accept the things I cannot change. I often joke that I am captain of the struggle bus.

If you know someone who is struggling with any battle, including cancer, I plea with you to remember the things you don't see. Silence can be the most telling of all when one is no longer strong enough for words. A kind gesture can go such a long way. We are so focused in our digital world that we often forget that sometimes human interaction is what someone may be missing the most in life. It is often the little things in life that mean the most.

34

Learning To Live Again

I have always needed purpose that resulted in the constant desire to make life easier for the ones who mean the most to me. It usually comes in the form of food from my love of baking and cooking, some sort of craft or a perfectly arranged gift basket. Since my diagnosis, I have lost some of the ability to take care of those closest to me, leaving me struggling with my purpose in life. If this last year has taught me anything, it is to embrace this new community that revolves around cancer, not the sadness, but the support and encouragement. I am surrounded by a tribe of women who understand every single trial I face without judgment. My family and friends are amazing, but this exclusive club offers me the one thing they are unable to provide me. I look forward to all I can offer in this new community with the hope that my experiences can help someone else who is struggling to know that they are not alone.

I continue to add travel experiences to my bucket list, filling stark white pages with colorful drawings and location ideas. We plan on spending more time at our second home in Florida. I intend to successfully make it through more concerts. I will fly to Ireland and Scotland one day with my husband. This man of mine has been a miracle with whom I will continue to create everlasting memories with. Love never quits. It weathers every storm and struggle together as one. My husband is my person, the one who both calms me as well as stirs my spirit. There will always be us.

I have succumbed to the fact there will be days my body refuses to cooperate, forcing me to reside in bed in order to rest and recover. Some days, I work on my digital scrapbook albums or write in my journal. When my joints allow it, I enjoy crocheting. It reminds me of my Mammy, who worked with a hook and yarn every day of her life, and keeps my hands busy from feverishly itching my chemo scalp. If I am too weak to do anything at all, then I watch television to catch up on my favorite series or an occasional Hallmark movie. Hanging beside my bedroom window are four grey wooden bars, each engraved with a different phrase, such as *Our Happy Place*. One piece holds five square metal photographs from Florida that include my sand castles, our fishing trophies as well as our memories on the water. They are full of bright colors of teals and blues that make me smile every time I look over that way from my bed. Our dresser holds a digital frame that rotates all of our Destin photos from our very first trip and beyond. I often find my husband standing over it watching them slide by as he reminisces of our trips there, making note of one snapshot of me that he finds extra special. These small mementos make my jello days a little brighter. I have an echo dot beside my bed that often shuffles my favorite playlists, whether it be reminiscing growing up in the eighties, relating to my inspirational songs, the usual country medley or the occasional old school hip hop. Music is good for the soul. It is often therapy providing relaxation as I get lost in the lyrics.

My chemo brain has made focusing on reading books difficult, much to my disappointment, as it has always been a pastime I enjoy. I began listening to audiobooks, which resulted in me having to teach myself to pay attention to it. After a few weeks, I was immersing myself in them daily whether I was curled up in my tower of plush pillows or cooking dinner. One book in particular was about a woman living with Leukemia that I could not stop thinking about in the weeks after completing it. I resonated with so much of her story being similar to my own. Shortly thereafter, I began writing my own narrative, unsure where it would take me, but hopeful it would also be therapeutic. I have never kept secrets from my husband, however, this was something I needed to keep to myself, hesitant if I would ever share my writings with anyone else. I worried they would think it was a terrible idea. Eventually, I shared the news with my family, who were, of course, both excited and supportive. My brother has published two novels, as well as an entire history book consisting of the genealogy from our father's side of the family. He also designed this amazing book cover for my story. Chad and I have both always been artistic with a fondness for photographs and artwork. As my writing began coming to an end, I decided to share my secret with my best friend and my cancer girls, who were beyond ecstatic for me, boasting how proud they were of this accomplishment. Writing this book was difficult for me, being someone who tries to portray that I am always fine while braving a smile. I have let my guard down to become vulnerable. I wasn't sure if I was going to let anyone read it, but the immediate positive response from my inner circle motivated me.

Some days it feels like I was just diagnosed yesterday, whereas, others it seems like I have always had cancer. I am working daily to let go of what I thought life would be, therefore creating a new path. My whole world was changed in a matter of minutes, which inevitably changed me. When I broke, I wanted to piece myself back together as the same person. That part of my life is in the past. I will rebuild myself better and stronger. It has given me more strength than I ever imagined I held within me. There have been times I have screamed, cried and fallen to the floor ready to give up. Sometimes, it's hard to get through the day, while other times are reminiscent of my pre-cancer life. I will always live in a daily reminder that I have cancer. The scar on my chest from my port will always be prevalent in the mirror, though someday I hope that reminder will fade away. Some days I am a warrior, while others I am a broken mess. I have learned to be calmer and to slow down a little. At the end of the day, I refuse to let cancer beat me down to someone I am not. Each and every time I fall, I will straighten up my crown and sparkle. The phrase "I'm fine" has been my safety net to hide behind over the last several years, but in reality, I AM fine. I am not alone. I have grown to accept that it is okay to not be okay all of the time. I have all the love and support I could ever ask for in my family, friends and my incredible medical team. They all have my best interest at heart and I will always be forever grateful for them. I have a strong faith to guide me. I am now part of an encouraging community that revolves around cancer. I hope that my story will inspire other survivors and caregivers and remind them that they are not alone in this fight. My brother tells me that my ordeal has made him a better, more compassionate, health professional. You can't truly understand life with cancer until you experience it yourself or through a loved one. Hopefully, my story has offered a small glimpse into that world for others.

There have been several new treatments and medications approved for Multiple Myeloma just in the last four years that I've been on this journey, along with many others that are still in the trial phase. I am confident that one day there will be a cure for not only my cancer, but all cancers that plague this world. I hope that I live to see the day that dream becomes a reality. Until then, I refuse to give up, continuing to make the best of this journey down the path I was given in this life, while filling my arm with another butterfly each year I celebrate yet another re-birthday.

Epilogue

My life will always be full of ups and downs riding the roller coaster that is Multiple Myeloma. I will go on to struggle with keeping my neutrophil count at an acceptable level and eventually give in to a few surgeries. My chemo regimen will continue to be ever-changing. Determined not to let those bumps in my path stop me, I look forward to crossing off all the adventures on my bucket list, starting with another concert.

We arrived to Youngstown, Ohio, surrounded by towering skyscrapers and clear blue skies. After checking into our hotel, we walked across the street to enjoy their wood fired pizza, margherita style, my favorite, layered with fresh mozzarella, thinly sliced tomatoes and fragrant green basil. We were diligent in spending some down time at the hotel so that I could rest a bit prior to the concert. Recently, I had been feeling a little better due to my chemo break in an attempt to allow my body to recover my immune system a bit. A yellow bicycle carriage seated in tufted black leather transported us over to the venue making the travel easier on my frail body. We found our seats next to the stage, strategically chosen on the back aisle, leaving nobody behind us. My husband was decked out in a thick caramel canvas vest and matte black cowboy hat, completed by chestnut boots. I wore an olive grey country t-shirt underneath a mustard sweater cardigan with a glamorous bling belt buckle.

The speakers began blaring with bright lights hovering over the enormous crowd. Phones were held high with their flashlights on, as concert goers swayed side to side.

We sang along to every song, exhilarated by the performance, and snapped several photos to commemorate the evening. As the night was coming to an end, the encore song began to play. It went straight to my heart, resonating so much with my life. Cody Johnson walked out to center stage to share his message:

"Take that phone call from your Momma

And just talk away

'cause you'll never know how bad you wanna

Until you can't someday.

Don't wait on tomorrow

'cause tomorrow may not show.

So say your sorries, your I-love-you's

'cause man you never know.

If you got a chance, take it,

Take it while you got a chance.

If you got a dream, chase it,

'cause a dream won't chase you back.

If you're gonna love somebody, hold 'em,

As long and as strong and as close as you can,

'til you can't.

The song came to an end as the crowd exploded with deafening cheers. Shawn kissed my lips, with a tear in his eye, smile across his face and said "You did it, baby." I had succeeded in enjoying another concert in a full arena. Later that evening, I curled up in the crest of his strong shoulder, happy and content. My husband kissed me on the forehead and whispered "One down, a million more to go." I purchased more tickets on our drive back home the next day.

"If you gotta chance, take it......"

Multiple myeloma is currently not curable, but we can manage the disease effectively for years. For active myeloma, treatment may include chemotherapy, proteasome inhibitors, immune-modifying drugs or other medications, or stem cell transplantation.

If this book has, in any way, touched your heart, I would humbly request that you visit www.themmrf.org and donate to the ongoing research being done to push back against this disease.

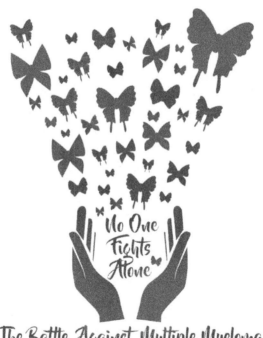

The Battle Against Multiple Myeloma

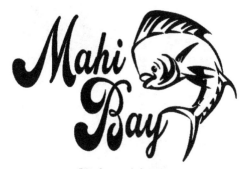

Okaloosa Island
Fort Walton Beach * Destin, Florida

If you are interested in viewing our condo:

www.airbnb.com/h/mahibayflorida

www.facebook.com/groups/mahibayflorida

Printed in the USA
CPSIA information can be obtained
at www.ICGtesting.com
LVHW091306141123
763825LV00005B/120